Y0-BTC-304

This book is destined to become the book on menopause. It provides the latest scientific information to empower women to cut through the confusion and make informed choices about nutrition, herbs, supplements and hormone replacement therapy. If you are entering or are already in menopause, this book is absolutely *Good for You!*

–JOEL M. EVANS, M.D.
FOUNDER AND DIRECTOR, THE CENTER FOR WOMEN'S HEALTH, DARIEN, CT
ASSISTANT CLINICAL PROFESSOR OF OB/GYN, ALBERT EINSTEIN COLLEGE OF
MEDICINE

A timely book written in the midst of the current HRT controversy facing women and confounding allopathic practitioners. Mary Ann Mayo presents an insightful, introspective compilation of facts from medical literature and evidence from clinical experience about women confronted with the physiologic changes of menopause/perimenopause. The book provides time-honored, safe alternatives to the risks associated with pharmacological estrogen and progestin use, and is well grounded in functional medicine research. Highly recommended reading for women of all ages.

–DAVID A. ELLIS, M.D., AAFP, ACAM

For every woman confused and frustrated with an avalanche of schizophrenic menopausal information, *Good for You!* is a thorough and compelling invitation to regroup, reassess and prepare for a spectacular second half of her life. From two women who have personally and professionally "walked the walk," this is practical advice rooted in sound science. This book should be required reading for all doctors who worship at the hormone altar.

–RANDY TOBLER, M.D.
ASSISTANT PROFESSOR OF OB/GYN
WASHINGTON UNIVERSITY SCHOOL OF MEDICINE
HOST OF *VITAL SIGNS* TALK SHOW

How refreshing! This book provides women the information and the tools to partner with their healthcare practitioners, empowering women to make balanced, educated choices about their treatment options! It is a realistic and motivating guide for women in taking personal responsibility for their self-care.

Understanding functional medicine (intercellular communication) and the availability of functional testing, coupled with critical thinking skills, should not be reserved for the relatively few of us who have made the commitment to this form of practice. *Good for You!* takes this essential approach to women's healthcare to the masses...at long last!

Thank you, Mary Ann and Lyra, for your commitment to educating and empowering women, as well as for your passion for communicating the intelligent healing capacity of the body.

—Dr. Lisa Perry
Doctor of Chiropractic, Clinical Practitioner and
Functional Medicine Consultant

Once again, Mary Ann Mayo has taken a distorted, confused and voluminous medical topic and made it informative, readable and applicable for women. Her sound and well-researched approach benefits medical professionals as well as the women to whom it is directed.

—Joseph L. Mayo, M.D., F.A.C.O.G.

Good for You! is a brilliant, process-oriented work filled with practical and provocative insights for both women and the practitioners who care for them.

Mary Ann Mayo and Lyra Heller emphasize the wisdom in a partnership of efforts, yet return the ultimate decision about hormone balance to each individual woman.

—Patricia H. Baldwin, R.N., M.S., N.P.
LifeSpan Women's Wellness

Refreshing! Mary Ann Mayo and Lyra Heller have written a how-to manual for every midlife woman struggling with the many changes that accompany menopause. Written in an engaging style, this manual encourages women to take responsibility for their health and to become informed partners with their healthcare providers.

—Ruth DeBusk, Ph.D., R.D.
Tallahassee, Florida

good for you!

by Mary Ann Mayo
with Lyra Heller

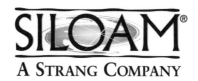
SILOAM®
A STRANG COMPANY

Most Strang Communications/CharismaHouse/Siloam products are available at special quantity discounts for bulk purchase for sales promotions, premiums, fund-raising and educational needs. For details, write Strang communications/CharismaHouse/Siloam, 600 Rinehart Road, Lake Mary, Florida 32746, or telephone (407) 333-0600.

Good for You! by Mary Ann Mayo with Lyra Heller
Published by Siloam
A Strang Company
600 Rinehart Road
Lake Mary, Florida 32746
www.siloam.com

This book or parts thereof may not be reproduced in any form, stored in a retrieval system or transmitted in any form by any means—electronic, mechanical, photocopy, recording or otherwise—without prior written permission of the publisher, except as provided by United States of America copyright law.

Unless otherwise noted, all Scripture quotations are from the King James Version of the Bible.

Cover design by The Office of Bill Chiaravalle | www.officeofbc.com

Author photo by Ron P. Jaffe

This book is not intended to provide medical advice or to take the place of medical advice and treatment from your personal physician. Readers are advised to consult their own doctors or other qualified health professionals regarding the treatment of their medical problems. Neither the publisher nor the author takes any responsibility for any possible consequences from any treatment, action or application of medicine, supplement, herb or preparation to any person reading or following the information in this book. If readers are taking prescription medications, they should consult with their physicians and not take themselves off of medicines to start supplementation without the proper supervision of a physician.

Author's Note: All references to clients in this book come from my clinical experience as a licensed marriage and family therapist working in a gynecologist's office. The cases I cite are composites of a number of clients who share similar issues and are equally protected with name and information changes to remain confidential. Any similarity between the names and stories of individuals described in this book and individuals known to readers is coincidental and not intentioned.

Copyright © 2003 by Mary Ann Mayo
All rights reserved

Library of Congress Cataloging-in-Publication Data

Mayo, Mary Ann.
  Good for you / Mary Ann Mayo.
    p. cm.
  ISBN 1-59185-170-X (pbk.)
1. Menopause—Hormone therapy—Popular works. 2. Menopause—Alternative treatment—Popular works. 3. Women—Health risk assessment—Popular works. I. Title.
RG186 .M337 2003
618.1'75061—dc21
2003014063

03 04 05 06 07 — 8 7 6 5 4 3 2 1
Printed in the United States of America

To Joe for his ability to give
To Lyra for her passion

Acknowledgments

Until 2002 definitive answers on the safety and use of hormones were not available. Nevertheless, the folks at Siloam, the health imprint of Strang Communications, have been keeping their eyes open for the newest solid information in their effort to make available truly cutting-edge work. Their encouragement, through the capable hands of Carol Noe, enabled me to bring forth a work free from preconceived or "alarmist-news" assertions. No pressure was applied for anything except a well-balanced, scientifically supported body of work that would help women sift through the claims, research and hype concerning their hormone health. Our mutual goal was to empower women to apply the *critical thinking skills* they use so well in other aspects of their lives to the selection of a health plan, practitioner and product.

Combined with Lyra Heller's years of experience, knowledge and commitment to wellness, we have accomplished what we set out to do—spelling out a "therapeutic lifestyle" plan that is scientifically responsible, reasonable to adopt and effective.

My personal effectiveness was enhanced by my husband, who suspended his world to see that I was fed, clothed and encouraged throughout this writing process. Not to be overlooked are his expertise and advice as a Stanford-trained obstetrician/gynecologist. I cannot adequately express how supportive he is—except to say all my women friends are envious!

good *for* you!

Contents

Part I: The Premise

Part II: The Baseline

Part III: The Action

Part IV: The Long-Term Perspective

PART I
The Premise

The need is real and urgent. You are on your own. While your physician works desperately to educate himself or herself on safe and effective alternatives to hormone replacement therapy or searches for the next "silver bullet," there is much you can do. Although the questions are many, and answers seem elusive, be assured—there are answers. You can decide what is good for you, given the right information. It may take a little work. But as a woman, you are used to work. It's just that it may seem new not to be spoon-fed when it comes to your health. Like anything new, it may feel awkward, but there is no question you are up to the task.

In these first chapters of Part I, you will be challenged to consider for yourself what is good for you.

Chapter one explores the dynamics of how the medical profession came to believe in a miracle cure with no definitive, scientific backing to demonstrate its efficacy.

Chapter two is the personal story of Lyra and me—a natural practitioner who cut her teeth on greens, or at least green medicine, and a therapist married to a Stanford-trained obstetrician/gynecologist.

Chapters three and four are meant to help you rethink the way you have traditionally approached the medical profession and the importance of getting beyond a "pill-for-an-ill" thinking.

And finally, chapters six and seven will build some new brain neurons as you examine your beliefs about menopause and aging, while learning how you can simply and safely influence your hormonal balance—and make smart choices for hormone health.

1

now what?

Physicians obligingly wrote forty-six million prescriptions for the hormone Premarin in its various components in the year 2000. With more than one billion sales in the United States, it was the second most frequently prescribed medication. It has been the leading hormonal choice of the medical profession for over fifty years. Premarin has weathered protests of the treatment of pregnant mares from which it is derived. It has survived the fact that a full 40 percent of women never filled their prescription for hormones and that more than half discontinued use within a year. But the announcement from the Women's Health Initiative reported in the summer of 2002 that combination hormone replacement therapy (HRT) did not convey the health benefits previously accepted by the medical community has taken its toll. There was an immediate drop in prescriptions by 40 percent—and that was just the beginning.[1]

Lest you think this is a problem for a handful of American women, consider these facts: It is estimated that there will be fifty million women entering menopause in the next few years. Each day forty-nine hundred boomer women start menopause, and there are millions of postmenopausal women, many of them hormone users for years.[2] One can hardly escape the aftermath. Go to the nearest coffee shop, gym or water cooler, and a cluster of women can be found personalizing and sharing their shock, despair, confusion and fear about hormone therapy. The most common questions are:

"What are you going to do?"

"What should I do?"

"What's next?"

The discussions continue for hours at times, while women cite situations of mothers, grandmothers and close friends, and conclusions vary:

"Just let them try and get my hormones away from me!"

"I quit cold turkey."

"I'm weaning off, but the hot flashes are keeping me up nights."

"I'm only taking them every three days."

"Well, I'm taking *natural* progesterone; do you think that is a problem?"

"I told you so. I told you to go to that clerk at the health food store; she has this stuff her sister makes that is all you need!"

It is no surprise that there are as many reactions and experiences as there are women.

Despite the varied opinions, when it comes right down to it, most women really *don't know* what to do. Especially disconcerting is the discovery that their doctors appear not to know either! After all, at their 2001 checkup they were told that if they refused to take hormones, they could plan on becoming the proverbial dried-up prune, humped over with osteoporosis and poised for a heart attack followed by a stroke. The only "good" news was that the decision *not* to take hormones would also result in loss of memory, so at least they wouldn't be aware of how bad off they were!

The 2002 checkup found many of those same doctors doing an about-face. HRT in one year had gone from a woman's salvation to a cancer-causing, stroke-producing trauma waiting to happen. It is a surprise that whiplash has not been added to the fallout of the list of problems with hormones!

The change of heart over hormones is not the only news that has undermined public confidence in the medical profession's recommendations. Controversy exists over the validity of regular mammograms, high-fiber diets and vitamin E for heart disease. Knee surgery for osteoarthritis has been declared ineffective. The new Cox-2 inhibitors and Vioxx advertised as "kinder, gentler" medications for arthritis have been found to cause ulcers just like the previous less-expensive versions. The government's food pyramid makes no sense to anyone, and, horror of horrors, just when you learned to cook a totally new way, you have been told you need fat in your diet after all. Just in whom and in what is a woman to put her faith?

It is clear that complete dependence on medical authority is not the choice. It never has been. Complete dependence on any authority is not a good idea. The pressure to surrender power to specialists in every field is a likely explanation and one of the major reasons why so many of us feel helpless. Doctors were never the clairvoyants we fantasized them to be. While some physicians may have reveled in such authority, most were painfully aware of the shortcomings of attempting to make a patient well without his or her participation and cooperation. Demanding that our physicians do for us what we were supposed to do ourselves makes wellness an illusive dream.

If a physician can't do it for us, can technology? This is the age of technology after all. Search long enough on the worldwide web, and answers will be found. Or will they? Apparently most of us missed class the day the teacher defined science as a *means of discovery*, not the source of definitive answers, especially ones that can be transformed into quick fixes for whatever ails you.

Still, our hope lies firmly rooted in the belief that quick fixes exist and that a wonder pill is out there to keep us in-line skating, acing *The New York Times* crossword puzzle, melting off those extra pounds and forever banishing hot flashes. All we need do, we daydream, is pick the miraculous formulary off the shelves of our local pharmacy.

That a quick fix might not exist is particularly rejected by baby boomers. They have no intention of contending with problems of aging. If the infamous "silver bullet" is not out there at the moment, it will be soon—so stay tuned. Their conviction disregards the reality that a whole generation of medical professionals, undergirded by technology, along with their female patients, believed in a pill deemed to be the ultimate silver bullet for millions of midlife women.

THE BREAKTHROUGH FROM THE BREAKDOWN

So here we are—our faith in the medical profession and technology shaken. The silver bullet turned out to be pot metal. Instead of hope lying in a one-size-fits-all pill for staving off the ills of aging, women face new and unfamiliar territory. Decisions must be made from a place that is untried, unplanned for, unimaginable and, if the truth be told, terrifying. But hold on; despite what it looks like, this isn't a crisis, a tragedy, the end of the world.

It is an opportunity. It is also a fleeting moment in time that may never come again. Already newer, shinier, silver bullets are being designed and tested. Doctors' prescription pads are only temporarily placed in the drawer. The crack in the omnipotent façade of the most highly developed medical system in the world grants us an opportunity to look behind the scene and see the scaffold holding everything up.

Was HRT ever really necessary? Its use can be compared to getting fitted for a pair of glasses. You go to the ophthalmologist because you have a problem seeing; otherwise, you would not choose to be fitted for glasses. You go to the gynecologist for HRT because you have a verifiable problem with hormone imbalance that requires hormones. Or, as is true for the majority, you go because of the prevailing belief that just being menopausal makes them essential. If you lose your glasses and cannot find someone to evaluate your eyesight and fit you for a better pair of glasses, you learn to live with your "new" vision. Your body's other senses are refined to compensate for diminished sight. Taste, touch, smell and hearing come to your rescue—automatically. Your world is interpreted through a "lens" not dominated by sight alone.

If you lose your hormone replacement therapy, in the same way, your body compensates—by adjusting to a gradual decline. Lower hormone levels are normal as we age, just as declining eyesight, hearing and the senses of touch, taste and smell are. However, there is a big difference between the ways we improve our senses—with glasses, hearing aids, special diets, supplements and specialized eye exercises—and the way we improve our hormone "balance." These "sense" remedies have no downside; the risk to benefit ratio is in favor of benefit. However, trying to remedy hormonal decline with HRT or in other ways has a risk factor that must be considered.

Adding hormones and wearing glasses are solutions to real problems of impaired function, but they are like comparing apples and oranges because one has little or no risk factor (wearing glasses), and the other (HRT) does. For sake of the analogy, your body adjusts to lowered hormones as it does to seeing without your glasses. This adjustment does not mean you are settling for less; it simply means you have the opportunity to explore, experience and explain reality with a different perspective than a twenty-year-old hormonally charged body. Do you dare to do so?

Good for You! is asking you to examine the scaffold of medical science that has been temporarily revealed and to take a chance on letting go of what has become too familiar. Peer through the crack. This breakdown is a *breakthrough*.

You have an unprecedented opportunity to examine what is *real*. It is natural to long for the quick fix; the drug model is the model of choice in America. While we should be grateful for the lifesaving medications that have contributed to greater wellness and health for young and old, we must also understand that medical interventions always involve a trade-off. Whether that trade-off is worth it—when to take the risk and how much of a risk it is—is at the heart of what this book is about. You need not fear it is all too complicated. The steps involved are ones mothers, wives and grown women of all persuasions use unconsciously all the time.

What to expect

We are going to make you aware of how you have already been acting and thinking like a scientist. You will become skilled at looking at interventions from the perspective of their risk/benefit profile. You will learn when to use a silver bullet. You will be fully aware of any trade-offs. You will discover that, more often than not, the body can be fixed without repercussion and further harm. You will become aware of how our culture uses pain, and you will understand the necessity of seeing beyond the agenda of eliminating it the quickest way possible. You will become a critical thinker.

WHAT COMES NEXT?

It is only fair that you know our destination. Lyra, my partner and researcher in this undertaking, and I want to have a conversation with you about being terrified when all you put your belief and trust in just went out the window. The issue is not simply whether the odds are in your favor for continuing or discontinuing hormone replacement. The much larger issue is how you came to believe that the quality of your future depended on maintaining hormonal levels your body naturally determines you no longer need in the doses you once did.

Accepting the challenge

Our first challenge and question is how we can ensure that you begin to think critically about *whatever* you decide to put into your body.

Our second objective is to confront the trepidation (terror) felt when you no longer believe you can know what is best for you.

Third, we need you to understand that everything you thought was real—*never* was. It is not the nature of science that everything is known and laid out in predictable ways. An appropriate use of science is to think like a scientist in determining a course of action and to develop an alternative plan when that doesn't work.

Fourth, you must develop a mind-set that considers risk/benefit when considering options available for healthful aging or relief of symptoms of menopause. We will share with you many options. We will make you aware of the ones that do not have the potential to cause harm. You may be less familiar with them, but they don't cause cancer or require adding additional pills to counteract side effects. We want to introduce you to them and let you use your critical thinking skills to discern what is best for you.

Fifth, we understand that you are operating under the folk adage: "Once stung, twice shy!" *Good for You!* is asking you to be "twice shy." You are rightfully cautious, suspicious and apprehensive about what is next.

At the same time, we want to help you see that this opportunity to look through the crack, to see things the way they really are, may never come again. It is appropriate to mourn the breakdown as long as the breakdown is seen as a breakthrough.

Sixth, it is important to understand how we got to a place where we believed that estrogen was a silver bullet. Unless you suffered from a clinical imbalance, the truth about hormones is that you more than likely never needed additional hormones at menopause in the first place. How did we all come to believe hormones at midlife were essential? Even the alternative medical community cast their vote for hormones—as long as they were "natural." The question to ponder is, "Who persuaded women they were sick and needed medicinal hormones?" When did you start to believe?

As you read, you are going to become a critical thinker in the area of your hormones. This book is not about giving you another silver bullet. There will be no claims made that any one intervention is a panacea. In other words, we are not going to give you the proverbial "fish"; we are going to teach you *how to fish*. But, never fear; we will not leave you without options. We will present what we know is helpful.

Anecdotal affinity

Lyra and I share menopause and aging with you. Our stories are unique, as is yours. I have been a writer on issues of women's health and in partnership with my Stanford-trained obstetrician/gynecologist husband in a medical clinic that specialized in menopause. Lyra Heller has for twenty years been the head herb developer and formulator for one of the largest natural supplement companies in America, a supplier of health practitioner's products and educational services in the area of complementary and alternative medicine (CAM).

Our differing life experiences nevertheless find us at a common juncture and sharing a mutual passion. We know you are already a scientist. We know you are the world's authority on you. We know you can discern a path that is right for you. We want to help you make it as risk free as possible. However, should your decision and/or particular health issues require intervention where risks are inevitable, we want your choice to be thoughtfully measured. And we want to introduce you to ways to approach your health issues that may be new to you.

Prevention: A "new" concept

The concept of prevention, making sure an individual doesn't get sick in the first place, is something doctors have rightfully been accused of knowing little about. For some physicians, if tests do not indicate a person is verifiably sick, there is little need for further involvement. But disease diagnosis is not prevention. New tests that measure how the body is functioning and pin-point early disease stages rather than the end stage are making inroads within the conventional medical community, but widespread acceptance is slow. So while science is changing, medical practice is not necessarily.

The scientific community is focusing more and more on refined ways to identify the presence of risk and the very early signs of tissue change. To be fair, it is difficult for an HMO, PPO or an individual medical practitioner to keep pace. So, new tests and more complex laboratory panels have to be fought for, as do innovative programs that support weight loss and provide education on nutrition and supplementation. And who will speak up for their addition? Chances are it will be you. Not because you have decided to become a medical crusader, but because you will know enough to demand the very best and safest care.

We are realistically faced with what to do when there is no silver bullet. Prevention and healing are equally important. Defining them anew is both the task and goal of this book. It is painful to have to acknowledge that keeping up on the latest, greatest quick fix is not the solution. It is a lot easier to take a pill than to learn how the body actually works—a forever-evolving story.

Our Creator designed a complex and brilliant system. When com-pleted, it was declared to be "very good" (Gen. 1:31). The magic and mys-tery of health lies not in the design of a miracle pill, but in the *design itself.* Good health involves restoring a perfect design.

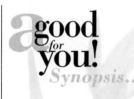

1. Can you see the seeming tragedy of hormone replacement therapy causing more harm than benefit as an opportunity for better health?
2. Is it prompting you to reevaluate your healthcare decisions?
3. Do you really believe there are valid, researched-supported ways to heal the body without causing it harm?

2

making it personal

I've always thought of myself as a healthy person. If you knew me, you would agree. I was very athletic in high school, thanks to my years in a Canadian school system that believed both boys and girls were capable of running and playing. I dabbled with gymnastics after college, desperate for something to do during those long hours my medical student husband was hitting the books. I picked up ballet again when I realized I envied my daughter's chance to wear a tutu and enjoy moving to great music. Until I was fifty, I was a dancing fool. I took up in-line skating following my sixtieth birthday; I started a yoga class at sixty-one years of age to keep my body flexible. Sometimes I even bound up my stairs.

My husband of forty years and I maintain an active social life. At quick glance I look good—healthy and well preserved—to be counted among the lucky ones. The American Association of Retired People (AARP) might even categorize me in *Modern Maturity* as the new image of aging. But looks can be deceiving, as the saying goes. I'm really not the picture of health I fantasize in my mind. In fact, I'm a mess. If I paid a dollar for every wrong thing going on in my body, I would probably not be able to buy groceries for the week. I suppose the real question or mystery, as the case may be, is why I appear to be in excellent health and why I continue to think of myself as healthy.

Indeed, given everything that is currently wrong or has been in the past, I should expect to be walking with a cane and doing crossword puzzles in bed. Even I am taken back when my personal image of myself as a healthy individual is forced to confront reality. (Maybe that is why I don't do it

8

often.) Honesty and a realistic assessment are demanded on the occasion of "breaking in" a new physician or facing the ordeal of filling out an insurance form—an act designed to make one sick.

My physical problems began at age five when, like thousands of others of my generation, I fell ill with polio. I happened to live in Houston, Texas, at the time. As my mother sat vigilantly by my bedside praying that the moving paralysis would not take up permanent residence, I recovered amidst the weekly gassing of the neighborhood with DDT—a factor that I believe contributed to other health problems as an adult. So as not to bore you, I will simply list my major health concerns.

---

onsider *this...* Polio at age five • Spondylolisthesis at age fifteen with episodes of major back pain throughout my twenties and thirties; hypoglycemia • At age twenty-six, six months of bed rest due to premature labor • At age thirty, multiple biopsies, precancer, bilateral mastectomy • At age thirty-one, reconstructive surgery with silicon implants • At age thirty-four, beginning of aches and pains, complaints of fatigue, mononucleosis, shingles, lactose intolerance, sinus infections, skin cancer (three squamous cells and several basal cells) • From age fifty to fifty-five, severe joint pain, fatigue, inability to exercise without excessive fatigue, surgery to remove what was left of the implants after more than twenty years, diagnosis of Hashimoto's thyroiditis, glaucoma • At age sixty, dry eye, cataracts, shingles, arthritis in hands and feet, postpolio syndrome.

I could also add to the list what I consider the longest menopause on record, but I admit my assessment is somewhat distorted. However, I still have hot flashes. Of all the things on that list, the most serious and the one with the greatest overall effect on my health is the series of lumps, bumps and mysterious precancerous entities that began cropping up in my breasts around my thirtieth birthday. While my aunt on my father's side was diagnosed with breast cancer late in life, my family is relatively cancer free. In order to maintain my only pregnancy, however, I had been confined to bed and was prescribed high doses of a progestin.

Five years later, I began to require biopsies every three months. Each time some new combination of cells would confound the pathologist and leave us completely confused. Eventually, it was decided that a subcutaneous mastectomy would be better than removing the breasts piece by piece. Despite my age I was all for such a decision. I reckoned that the next biopsy or the next would reveal full-blown cancer, and then I really would have something to worry about. The pathologist agreed. We had a five-year-old, and my husband and I had just adopted a baby girl.

Reconstructive implants were barely being discussed at the latest surgical meetings. Still, I was at peace with what for many is an inconsolable loss. The options seemed clear to me: Have the surgery and live, or wait another couple of years until cancer was diagnosed, have the surgery and probably die. I was happy to have a choice. The loss of both breasts seemed a minor exchange for the privilege of seeing my kids marry and growing old with the man I loved. I still feel that way.

What I didn't expect was the impact the decision made to "look normal" would have on the rest of my life. My surgeon approached me six months after the mastectomy and suggested that I might consider placement of the new silicon implants into what was essentially two holes in my chest, which for lack of anything better, I occasionally filled with my husband's socks. You might think that I would have jumped at the chance, but I didn't. If I truly believed I was the same person with or without breasts, why would I consider replacing them with imposters? It was the height of the women's movement after all, and enlightened women cared about such issues!

The decision to have the surgery came down to practicalities. Getting clothes to fit would be easier, but most importantly, my newly adopted daughter would have one less concern in life; her mommy would look like everyone else's. Only secondarily did I hesitate because of health concerns. "Would they break?" I asked. "What if I was in a car wreck and hit the steering wheel?" I was quickly assured that since silicon was "inert," there would be no health sequelae other than flaunting perky breasts some day in an old folk's home.

But there were health repercussions. For years I denied the connection. Even though we were in the medical profession, not one of our colleagues saw a correlation between silicon implants and the fatigue, joint pains and general malaise I was increasingly suffering. I had excuses for my deteriorating health. I was a driven type A; the name of the game was to "carry on," preferably at record pace.

As the years rolled by, each annual physical began with complaints of fatigue. By the time I was fifty my joint pains were intense, but don't all dancers ache? Our move to northern California was motivated in part by our desire to reduce stress and improve my health. Instead, I continued to decline; we estimated I would be unable to get around on my own within five years. Consequently, we began constructing a house that would accommodate a wheelchair.

By then Connie Chung had opened Pandora's box with her exposé on breast implants. Attendance at meetings in which rooms full of women shared my complaints overcame any doubts that many of my problems were related to silicon. Twenty years had passed since my surgery, and it was a well-accepted fact that silicon did not stay confined within its outer shell and almost immediately began to "weep" through the silicon casing. I made the decision for their removal. And for me, wearing prosthesis is easy compared to living with what I felt had become a toxic minefield on my chest.

something *to* *think about*

Not all women who have silicon implants have health problems. Not everyone is allergic to nuts, but those who are can react mildly or have life-threatening emergencies. Genetic propensity and previous toxic exposure are among the factors that make the difference.

My goal in having the surgery was to halt the deterioration of my health. I had no expectation of getting better. But, miraculously, I did. I credit both my God, in His infinite wisdom, who prompted us to move to an area in the heart of alternative medicine gurus, as well as the brilliant men and women we met there. They reminded us of the perfect design of a body working as it was meant to, teaching us how to return it to that state. I share my story because it explains how a conventionally trained physician became a practitioner of integrated (functional) medicine. My husband's most passionate speech is entitled, "What I Didn't Know About Medicine Almost Cost Me My Wife."

There is no greater argument for accepting a new approach to healing than when someone you love has found renewed health and vitality. I continue to deal with autoimmune illnesses such as Hashimoto's thyroiditis and arthritis, most likely set in motion by the many years my body fought a toxic exposure (perhaps beginning with DDT while fighting a serious disease as a child). Yet, I maintain a sense of wellness by focusing on activities, nutrition and supplements and some conventional interventions that maximize the way my body is supposed to work. I am also increasingly aware that my sense of well-being is attributable as well to the personal bias I hold about myself that *I am a healthy person and the things I do to feel better will work.*

I have experienced firsthand that a "functional" approach to health provides optimal wellness for me and that my attitude plays a part, regardless of the difficulties I must face. I am not disease or problem free, and I never will be. But I am able to live my life doing almost everything I want or need to do.

BUT WHAT ABOUT MENOPAUSE?

As Lyra shared with me her personal *one-month* menopause experience, I wasn't sure whether to look at her with a renewed awe or whack her on the side of the head. By contrast, I became aware of menopausal changes around age forty-two. I began waking up at night sweating and wondering why the room had suddenly gotten so hot. Months passed before I made the connection that I was having night sweats as the result of hot flashes. However, my real concern was the abrupt change in my memory. I could not recall ordinary words. "That is such a pretty uh…uh, well you know, uh…jacket," I would stumble out. I began to panic. There is not a person alive who does not have a "worst-fear" scenario—mine is that I will lose my mind.

Since my childhood, being able to think, study and learn has been a personal value. I was never at the top of my class, but I so admired those who were. I studied hard and obsessed over tests despite my mother's admonition to "calm down." I dismissed such advice, choosing instead to become a perfectionist—a defeatist ideology since nothing one does is ever good enough. When my mother developed Alzheimer's disease and her twenty-three years of diminishing synapses took her from me, my own worst fear intensified. It reached neurotic proportion until this year, when I set aside the time to write a book about my fears, *Twilight Travels With Mother* (Fleming Revell, 2003), developing a proactive strategy for those of us who are convinced that losing our mind is just around the corner. My fear prompted me to accept the invitation to write this book as well. I figured I had better do it while I could.

"Just *do* something!"

While I have become aware of the esteem I hold for a well-functioning cerebellum, how that influenced my medical decisions remained largely unconscious and unexamined. I could deal with hot flashes by opening the bedroom windows and wearing light nightclothes, but nothing I did seemed to improve my mind. My periods were regular, and my hormone levels only barely reflected my age, but I was desperate to stop my eroding memory. I approached my bewildered husband and demanded he do something. After all, he was the gynecologist; I was just the melancholic female.

Consistent with his training, he suggested I try hormone replacement therapy (HRT). I was willing to do anything if it promised I might hold on to even one synapse. And miraculously it worked. Within three weeks it was as if someone had turned on a light bulb in my brain. I was ecstatic. The fact that I was so willing to take HRT despite my mastectomy (and warnings against it being given to anyone who has experienced cancer) is a measure of how important a keen mind was to me.

A fear synergy

There is one other menopausal experience, this one coming years later, that is equally worth telling. As sometimes happens, hot flashes come and go, and their intensity varies. I experienced one month in which a hot flash would reach its peak, begin to ebb and then head back up the charts again— wave upon wave, one after another. Before they stopped (as mysteriously as they had begun), I reached a place of pure despair and was flirting with panic. As I recalled this incident with Lyra, we began to explore why I found that episode so alarming. At first I rhapsodized about the physical misery, then the connection was made that the real problem was my old one. The intensity and duration of my flashes had become distracting enough that I was not able to think. So, it wasn't the raging heat I couldn't bear; it was the fear of an unavailable mind.

Hopefully you are more aware of the platform from which you are making your health decisions. If not, it is a valuable exercise to review your medical history with the overlay of your personality and family or the life-time influences that are the nidus (seedbeds) of your decision making.

From another world

Lyra Heller is one of those *brilliant* people I referred to that helped us learn a new way of practicing medicine. Much of her appeal lies in her all-encompassing approach to life and the passion, which is always a part of what she does. The synergy between us feeds us both. Neither one of us would have attempted this book without the other.

Lyra's story is very different from mine. Her background for three generations has been in the alternative medical community. I doubt that the word *fatigue* is part of her vocabulary, and I'm sure it has never appeared as part of her medical history. Amazingly, with the exception of childhood illnesses, she has never been sick. There have been the occasional cold or flu bugs. But they left within seventy-two hours seeking someone more vulnerable after deciding Lyra's body was far from a prime "growth medium," as they say in laboratories. Her body has remained slim pickings for germs despite the fact that she has never been vaccinated and, with three minor exceptions, has never used antibiotics. Did I say she has never taken an aspirin? Well, maybe three times in her fifty-six years, following dental work and once with an extremely high adult fever when homeopathic remedies were not available.

Of course, Lyra didn't set out to be the healthiest little girl around; it was her father's idea, a chiropractic doctor. She was exempt from the usual preschool injections on religious grounds. As a result she caught the German measles in her twenties and shared the chicken pox with her son. Her only serious brush with the conventional medical profession occurred two years ago when a small speck turned up on a mammogram. The biopsy that followed was benign.

Lyra didn't have to acquire an interest in natural (physical or green) medicine; she grew up unaware that other options existed or, more accurately, that nothing else could be trusted. If she got a cold, the family's choice of remedy was a specially prepared extract of Irish moss, along with increased vitamin C, for example. She had no experiences with conventional doctors whose training advocates giving a "pill for an ill," which means, more precisely, prescribe a strong medicine like an antibiotic for a commonplace, self-limiting complaint like a cold or flu, or a nonsteroidal anti-inflammatory drug (NSAID) for back pain, a strain or sprain. Lyra's childhood medicine was an herb, a homeopathic remedy, a chiropractic adjustment, a massage or a faith healer who would lay hands on her. The tools used to get rid of symptoms shared an underlying philosophy and strategy that addressed and removed obstacles to health, allowing the body to heal itself.

Fortunately for Lyra, her father's approach included a great deal of common sense. She was taught that not all natural products were safe. It was important that she learn how to use them responsibly and respectfully—a characteristic she applies today as procurer and formulator of natural products.

What her father's medicine didn't teach was that emotions might have something to do with health; there was no mind/ body model from his perspective. A physical model of medicine precluded questions being asked about lifestyle or the mind/emotional component of a patient's life.

Lyra points out that while reverence was reserved for the body's ability to heal itself, her childhood learning was taking place amidst "crazy-making," emotional family scenarios. One Christmas when she was five years old, she awoke to find a new doll house and a complete stranger in their kitchen. Without much explanation, she and the stranger boarded the Red Line electric bus system in operation in Los Angeles at the time and made their way across town to a hospital room where her mother was being prepped for surgery.

Amidst a confusing flurry of activity and great emotion, just as her mother was about to be wheeled from the room, Lyra's father picked her up and, her robe flying in the wind, carried her to their car for the trip home. Years would pass before she saw another conventional physician. Her mother was told she had lymphoma and would die within months. She did eventually die of cancer, years later—from breast cancer—when she was in her sixties. The nine siblings of her mother all died of cancer. None were involved with alternative health and all lived fairly long lives. You should not be surprised to learn that Lyra's biggest health concern is breast cancer.

At this juncture, neglecting his practice, Lyra's father began to make his life's work that of keeping her mother alive. So Lyra grew up with the desire to be healthy, using physical medicine, characterized by giving the body the nutrients it needs, with the application of human physiology principles. Physical medicine is based on the premise that specific foods are medicine, homeopathy is medicine, herbs are medicines—and that the diet a person eats becomes medicine by intention. What she didn't learn, as we mentioned, was how and where the mind and spirit were supposed to intersect.

But for Lyra, from age eight until she was thirty-five years old, an odyssey began in which her mother went in and out of remission at least nine times. Her healthy and sick times were remarkably timed to coincide with family crises, including unpopular choices her only daughter, Lyra, would occasionally make. Lyra watched as the destructive power of anger undid for her mother the times of seemingly miraculous healing. She saw the power of the body at work. It became evident to Lyra that maintaining good health involved more than simple manipulation of the food you eat.

Her father had nothing good to say about conventional practitioners. Nevertheless, he and her mother insisted that Lyra become one. She was to take care of them and fulfill their desire for her to become, in her words, "the biggest, most important regular doctor in the whole wide world." The peril of not doing so was to cause her mother to become sick again—with the awful possibility of feeling she would be the one to cause her mother's death.

Needless to say, Lyra's decision to enter graduate school to study anthropology instead of attending medical school was a life-defining moment. But, having lived with the dynamics of illness so closely coupled with emotion, her passion was to study how societies on a worldwide scale confront and live with illness. She wanted to understand what human nature has to do with the origin of illness and how the mind is involved with destructive, guilt-inducing patterns that cause physical harm.

In school she confronted her bias that Western medicine is bad and natural medicine is good. She concluded that both systems could stand side by side and live by the creed "to do no harm." She has chosen to keep another acknowledged bias, the one declaring that the body is capable of healing itself. But she is adamant that stimulating the body to come back into balance requires the reexamining of all traditional medical systems used throughout the generations. There are commonalities that Western medicine tends to ignore. This current HRT crisis, for example, is an open door to reevaluation, giving enlightened conventional physicians new motivation and opportunity to reevaluate medical systems they have previously dismissed outright.

Good for You! thinking

Lyra believes strongly that individuals can be helped to reason, think clearly and focus analytically on the pros and cons of options available for healing. She is an advocate of *critical thinking,* thinking like a scientist. The core for her approach, like her father's, remains focused on foods: healthy food to feed the body and concentrated, specially prepared versions for illness. Unlike her father, her integrative approach requires consideration of mind and body. What affects one affects the other.

Lyra states, "I came to understand that how one chooses to live with people in relationship has as much to do with healing as choosing which herb you use. The discomfort felt when you are looking for new treatments must include exploring pieces from the past, finding the 'blind spots,' if you will, that prevent you from living a fully expressed life. The restraints and obstacles to healing can be beliefs you blindly adopted from people you respect— without making a conscious choice. They may result from feelings of resentment, anger or fear, which appear buried, but that direct your choices twenty-four hours a day. To feel love and not express it can be just as damaging as to harbor resentment."

something *to* *think about*

To feel love and not express it can be just as damaging as to harbor resentment.

—Lyra Heller, 2003

Struggling with personal bias

Lyra confesses that in her struggle with the fear of cancer, she is tempted not to embrace conventional medicine, although she knows, intellectually, that is unwise. She forced herself to get a DXA (a test for measuring bone density) and a mammogram but has let two years go by without a follow-up, despite its revelation of a small benign spot. Her "unexpressed" assumption (until recently) has been, "I will die of cancer, and I can't do anything about it." The phenomenon of menopause, however, has wrought its mysterious transformation and has given her the courage to face the possibility she can change her destiny.

Now she declares, "I am a candidate for cancer, but I am working on a more positive attitude by uncovering blind spots I wouldn't look at before—like acknowledging that not practicing what I preach affects my husband and family deeply and what I do really matters to the people I love." From a practical standpoint, for the first time she is seriously confronting the extra pounds that increase her cancer risk. She has been successful by thinking one day at a time and finding encouragement from short-term markers that measure success.

While there is no way to prove it, her lifetime practices likely explain the ease with which she has gone through menopause. She is the poster child for our premise that the healthier you are when you enter the change, the easier it will be. Her biggest worry had been when it would happen. Her hopes for an early menopause (which is associated with a lower breast cancer risk) were dashed as it wasn't until she reached the age of fifty-five and one-half that she missed her first period. Her first hot flash was experienced while lecturing in front of one hundred people. She didn't recognize it at first, but her audience delicately reminded her that its origin was not the result of a hot room.

This year (2003), at age fifty-six, periods stopped and severe flashing began on a fifteen-minute cycle. She began using soy isoflavones, vitamins, minerals, fish oils and a special selection of antioxidants, and after two weeks they were reduced to one per hour. After five weeks, they came approximately one every two hours, then slowly disappeared. Thus her menopause discomfort essentially lasted around two months.

And what about you?

Now you know our stories, in part. What about yours? True confessions are never easy. It takes courage to look into your story. Within it are biases and assumptions that have influenced your health choices as well as your attitude about menopause. To use this book to your advantage, you need to begin to explore what they are. While a general draft will come to mind rather quickly, keep your mind open to additional data that are likely to filter into your consciousness in the weeks ahead.

There is a need to allow the unconscious to become conscious. You may have gone your entire life not realizing the opportunities and choices that are possible. An awareness of your story will be a factor in the decisions you make about medical and alternative options that will be presented. Our goal is to ensure you are aware of the factors that go into your decision making so that ultimately what you decide to do is right for you, effective and healthy in the long term. Obviously, the more you understand the way your body works, the more likely you will make decisions consistent with what it needs.

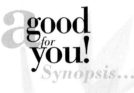

1. Identify the conscious and unconscious biases and assumptions at work relative to your health and menopause.

2. How were medical crises handled in your family of origin?

3. How do you ensure the safety of your medical choices?

4. Is being disease free the only way you can be healthy?

5. Do you believe on some level that you can abuse your body and escape the consequences?

3

the rest of the story: a new medicine for now

Once upon a time there was a beautiful midlife woman. Her eyes were bright, anticipating all that lay ahead; her heart was filled with a joy she shared with anyone with whom she came in contact. Since retiring from her teaching job, she filled her days volunteering at a local welfare store whose funding supported underprivileged youth. Quality time was allotted for taking care of friends whose illnesses required her tender touch, good cooking and adeptness with bedpans. There was time for her husband of over thirty years, Alphie the cat and the flowers she nurtured on her deck.

One day a black cloud appeared right over her house. Its ominous presence matched the gloom with which her once cheery continence was covered. She didn't feel good. She had been uncharacteristically irritable and so very tired. When her sick friend needed her, she had to fake her willingness to once again drop by. She lashed out at her husband when he innocently asked what her plans were for dinner. And, wouldn't you know it, it was time to take Alphie to the vet. To make matters even worse, the new volunteer worker at the store, who at first seemed to be someone who would share the load, was becoming more trouble than help. It was all too much. She started to cry and found she couldn't stop.

Now, "beautiful midlife woman" was smart enough to know that something was very wrong. Let's follow three scenarios of what she might do next.

ACT 1, SCENE I: THE VISIT WITH DOCTOR USUAL

"Beautiful midlife woman," hereafter known as *BMW*, did the responsible thing and made an appointment with her doctor. The nurse took her blood pressure. It was high: 140/90. She was surprised to see she had gained another ten pounds since her previous visit. Dr. Usual was his *usual* friendly self. He listened carefully as she explained her increasing fatigue and nightly awakenings. She also shared that she was moody and sensed a difference in her ability to handle stress.

Dr. Usual perused her chart and asked if a previous yeast infection she had called in about had cleared up. BMW reported that it had and that she had added yogurt to her diet, which seemed to have reduced its occurrence. She thought she detected a slight rolling of Dr. Usual's eyes, but she chose to give him the benefit of the doubt. Dr. Usual counseled her on her activities, suggesting that she become less involved, start walking daily and "watch" her weight gain. Looking at his watch, he wrote a prescription for a diuretic medication and reminded her that if her sleep problems continued, he would refer her to a new sleep clinic for evaluation. He put his arm on her shoulder with what seemed like genuine caring, wished her well and called his next patient. The nurse reassured her there was no need to make another appointment but to feel free to call if she needed to. BMW left unsure if the visit had been worth the time she had spent, but dutifully stopped by her pharmacist and filled her prescription.

Act 1, Scene 2

A year later, at BMW's annual checkup, Dr. Usual was pleased to find that BMW's blood pressure had dropped to slightly above the normal range. She had lost ten pounds and was sleeping somewhat better. Her fatigue and general sense of wellness were much worse, but they seemed so nebulous BMW didn't bother to mention them again. This time she was given a prescription for statins (medicine that lowers cholesterol) in response to the results of her blood test and her high lipid panel.

ACT 2, SCENE 1: A VISIT WITH DR. UNUSUAL

BMW had never been to Dr. Unusual before. She was surprised when his receptionist asked her to reserve an hour and a half for the first visit. She was told to expect a packet of information in the mail that she needed to complete and return before her actual visit. BMW was not thrilled; she had enough to do, especially when she realized that the paperwork required filling out a number of rather extensive questionnaires, as well as detailed information about her own and her family's health. But, having a teacher's heart, she diligently did as much as she could.

The nurse weighed BMW and, as she stepped off the scale, slipped a measuring tape around her waist. BMW blushed but decided not to say anything. Her blood pressure was noted, and she was escorted into Dr. Unusual's office. He was pleasant, beginning the conversation by asking if she missed teaching and how she filled her days. He had clearly read the material she had sent in; he asked for clarification on several points and discussed the relevance of her answers to some of the questionnaires.

He explained that the combination of symptoms she was experiencing—her weight gain, sleeplessness and fatigue—made him suspect she might be suffering from hyperinsulinemia or perhaps even metabolic syndrome, also known as Syndrome X. This was news to BMW. From her perspective, she was "fat," and everyone knows how that happens. Dr. Unusual gave her some information to take home and read. He explained her pancreas could be working overtime to produce high levels of insulin that her body was not using effectively. Insulin is supposed to transport glucose, the fuel her cells need for energy production. He suspected her cells were failing to respond, a condition called "insulin resistance." As a result, her body had difficulty burning calories and she likely had increased blood sugar levels and muscle loss. If tests revealed high cholesterol and triglyceride levels along with her elevated blood pressure, Syndrome X was likely— a combination of factors that put an individual at high risk for heart disease, stroke, diabetes and Alzheimer's.

Dr. Unusual noted that her expanding waistline had reached proportions that increased her cardiovascular risk. Before making recommendations, he wanted her to have a number of baseline tests. The results would be considered in light of her family history and current routines. At that point he would suggest some therapeutic lifestyle interventions and evaluate her diet and supplement use. He recommended that she immediately make time for a daily walk. It would serve as a sleep aid, release stress, help her lose weight and improve her cardiovascular and Alzheimer's risk profile. She was sent to the lab and asked to return in one week.

Act 2, Scene 2

BMW did manage to walk four times the following week and had to admit to Dr. Unusual that it seemed that one simple intervention had helped her feel better. Dr. Unusual was encouraging, but disclosed that her conventional testing (lipids, two-hour postchallenge glucose and insulin level test, homocysteine, C-reactive protein) was suggestive of Syndrome X.

To gain further information, he requested that she take an adrenocortex stress profile test, which was unlikely to be covered by her insurance. The results of this noninvasive assay would measure her levels of DHEA (dehydroepiandosterone) and twenty-four-hour (circadian) rhythm of cortisol, hormones that affect anxiety, fatigue, obesity and diabetes among other chronic diseases. It was a test that measured *function* rather than *pathology*. Among other things, it would provide valuable information that could be used to improve her sleep pattern. BMW agreed.

Dr. Unusual explained that before he would recommend medications that might reduce some of her risks but increase others (like statins and blood pressure medication), he wanted her to begin therapeutic lifestyle interventions. He assured her that nothing he suggested was harmful. He was adamant that she increase her walking—exercise reduces insulin resistance.

Rather than tell her to "watch" her weight, as Dr. Usual had done, she was given a video that explained how the production of insulin is triggered by some foods more than others. If her diet continued to be one of high glycemic foods, her body would generate more insulin, and she would continue to feel hungry faster and store more fat. She was to include "good" fat and avoid "bad" fat. High-quality, portion-controlled protein accompanied by carbohydrates in the form of vegetables, fruit and whole grain could improve her lipid profile while helping her lose weight. For three months she was to report weekly to Dr. Unusual's staff nutritionist to monitor progress and have questions answered.

The nutritionist helped BMW choose supplements that were foundational and add extra formulations that were helpful for improving her metabolic imbalance and her lipids. The addition of Guggulipid (an herbal extract) played a role in reducing her total cholesterol and LDL.

After the results of the *adrenocortex stress profile* were returned, Dr. Unusual directed BMW through a program to adjust her sleep patterns. To reduce stress he encouraged her to prioritize her time, leaving room for activities that were restorative. He insisted she take a yoga exercise class. She was reluctant to add anything to her schedule, so she was pleased that her yoga instructor helped her put together at-home exercises for deep breathing, stress relief and stretching. After several months of class, she was confident and motivated enough to maintain an at-home routine that only took her ten or fifteen minutes, which she followed with a time of prayer.

After one year, BMW lost thirty pounds without dieting, felt revitalized and found her new therapeutic lifestyle not only returned her sense of joy, but it also gave her greater energy and verve to face each day. She no longer had trouble sleeping and had measurably reduced her risk factors for heart disease and diabetes.

Now consider what might have happened if BMW's visit to Dr. Usual had been after reading *Good for You!* Could you do what she does in the following scenes and motivate your "Dr. Usual" to become a "health partner"?

ACT 3, SCENE 1: A REMATCH WITH DR. USUAL

BMW made an appointment with Dr. Usual, who listened but didn't address her complaints, other than telling her she must reduce her stress, lose weight and fill the prescription he was giving her. BMW spoke up. She has read a book called *Good for You!* and has become a critical thinker. She memorized the chapter on talking to your doctor (see chapter nine) and is clear about what she wants.

"Before I go, doctor," she said respectfully, "I would like you to order some basic laboratory tests that will include a lipid panel, thyroid and glucose." She continued, "You see, I'm concerned I might have some insulin resistance—and looking in the mirror, I see I could be a candidate for Syndrome X." Dr. Usual's eyes glazed over. He coughed, and BMW noticed a slight tinge of red rising from his color. She was aware her hands had become sweaty. She took a deep breath. Dr. Usual picked up his pen and began to write rather furiously. BMW wondered if he was making a note to himself, something like: "Note to nurse: When BMW calls for an appointment, tell her I've moved to Caney Creek, Oklahoma." Instead, he looked up, smiled and replied, "Well, I don't think so, but if it sets your mind at ease, let's do that."

Emboldened by her success, there was no stopping BMW. "Dr. Usual, while you are at it, add on the adrenocortex stress profile. It might give us some insight into my sleep issues and fatigue before you send me to the sleep clinic." Dr. Usual sensed there was no need arguing. "Tell me about this test," he said. BMW deftly placed an information sheet in his hands pointing out the credentials and location of the laboratory, its FDA approval and a direct phone line for physicians. He cautioned her that she would most likely have to pay for the test herself, although they were both pleasantly surprised when her insurance covered the cost.

Act 3, Scene 2

When the laboratory tests results were in, BMW and Dr. Usual discussed them, agreeing that in combination with her family history it did look as if Syndrome X was a likely possibility. Dr. Usual agreed to monitor her therapeutic lifestyle steps for three months to see if the pattern improved. If not, she agreed to begin some pharmaceutical interventions. Without the help of a nutritionist, BMW had to educate herself over the Internet on sound nutritional practices, and she began to adjust her eating habits. She ensured she got enough exercise by pushing her ailing friend in her wheelchair.

Deciding on a supplemental regimen proved difficult. Dr. Usual seemed suspicious of all supplemental support, citing the risk involved. BMW thought that was interesting, considering his willingness to give her pharmaceutical drugs with a much higher risk profile. She rejected her friend's multi-marketing solution and bought a couple of books by reputable authors at the local health food store. She studied and made her selections, using criteria that included understanding why she was taking each product and assurance that they were made by trustworthy companies. In three months, follow-up tests indicated that her interventions were leading her in the right direction. Even Dr. Usual conceded that nothing she was doing appeared harmful. He acted even friendlier than "usual" toward her.

Act 3, Scene 3

BMW vacillated between wishing someone would just tell her what to do and basking in the increased control and power she felt. With each visit, Dr. Usual became more of a health partner. Pushed by an intelligent patient, he appeared increasingly motivated to learn and incorporate an overall approach to healing the body versus his previous singular focus on symptoms. BMW is now happy to recommend him to her friends as "someone who will work with you." Her medical care is, if not perfect, at least giving her a sense of control, helping her feel better and, mysteriously, leaving her with a sense of peace.

Who knows? As fate would have it, Dr. Usual and Dr. Unusual could one day find themselves sitting together at a medical meeting. Dr. Usual might prove open to further changes in his fundamental philosophy of practicing medicine. That he was open to BMW's suggestions is really not so surprising. If you recall, it was the baby boomers who changed the practice of obstetrics by demanding natural childbirth and that they share the birthing experience with their husbands. Currently, they are putting pressure on physicians to reconsider their "one-note" approach to menopause. Never underestimate the power of a woman to change a whole medical system!

THE CONVERSION OF DR. USUAL

Just what is Dr. Usual missing? He is a graduate of a terrific medical school and has a genuine heart to help people. He is able to rise to the call when acute illnesses are the issue, and his skill and knowledge have saved lives. Isn't that valid criteria for a medical career? Why then are his methods so unsatisfactory for prevention and treatment of degenerative and/or chronic diseases—the everyday aches and pains and general malaise of not feeling well?

Or, maybe you are more curious about Dr. Unusual? It should ease your mind to know that Dr. Unusual is not someone who is a figment of this writer's imagination. He, or she, is out there, and there are more like him. Why is he different? What factors kept him from looking at BMW as a "pill-for-an-ill" candidate? Dr. Unusual is likely to have graduated from the same medical school as Dr. Usual, but at a given point, his interests diverged. We can only speculate, but perhaps he got tired of seeing how ineffective "medicine as usual" was for long-term illnesses and general well-being. Somewhere along the line he became convinced that not getting sick in the first place was preferable to efforts at curing—a goal perhaps shared with Dr. Usual but pursued more earnestly by Dr. Unusual, who is aware he has power to make a difference.

Chances are someone Dr. Unusual loved or worked hard to care for didn't respond to all he had learned at the best medical school or from the latest journal. There were things in medicine he didn't know how to fix despite great knowledge and expertise. His response was not to give up on conventional medicine and all its bells and whistles, but to search for ways to have a better outcome. Whether it was by accident or design, he was open to finding other ways to approach healing. Ironically, most are based on old traditions. In order to practice medicine successfully and do no harm in the process, he had to look at the body in its totality while simultaneously utilizing the very latest technology for understanding the inner working of each individual and how the information obtained meshed with the external.

Good medicine

Dr. Unusual's brand of medicine is not alternative medicine or conventional medicine with a twist. It is *good medicine*. If it must be categorized, it is a *functional* medicine approach. This is different from the emphasis he learned in medical school. There, Drs. Usual and Unusual learned how to relieve symptoms. They were tested on underlying causes of symptoms; they heard little about prevention of the underlying causes. More accurately, what was taught about underlying causes did not take on significance when compared with treating symptoms and making someone feel good again as quickly as possible. Besides, these medical students were told that a sure way to become discouraged was to depend on the patients' diligence to follow a program that required them to be responsible for improving their health, rather than simply receiving the magical elixir from the professional.

"Officially" sick

A by-product of the emphasis on symptomology (treating symptoms of disease rather than cause) is the development of laboratory tests that measure the point at which you officially have a disease. Almost every test Drs. Usual and Unusual learned to interpret in medical school did not teach them how well an organ or organ system functioned. It was designed to diagnose disease—you have it or you don't. You are sick or you are well. But, you insist, "I feel terrible!"

One of two things is likely to happen should your tests declare there is no reason for you not to be out conquering the world or running a marathon. One, you may be subjected to more tests. Two, you will be dismissed (nicely) with the secret word *m* for *malinger* (one who pretends to be ill) in the lower right-hand corner of your doctor's notes. Well, perhaps not, but it feels that way. When test results cannot be easily explained or quantified in some way, there is a tendency to dismiss or overlook a patient's complaints.

The truth is, many clinical and personal experiences fall outside the established "norm," operate under natural law or are to be found within the parameters of human spirituality. When you feel bad but your tests essentially call you a liar, it is hard to decide where to direct your anger. For most patients it circulates between the dog, the spouse, the doctor and themselves! Sometimes, judging by the numbers, there is a simple solution when tests fail to indicate anything is wrong yet a patient is insistent. It is, of course, a prescription for the handy, dandy, all-purpose fixer-upper—Prozac, Paxil or the like.

Consider *this…* If good medicine is defined as treating the cause of a problem rather than the symptom, how does today's medical practice stack up?

WHY FUNCTION LOSES OUT TO SYMPTOMS

It is a health practitioner's calling to relieve suffering. It is an easy transition from this medical charge to a sincere belief that if there is pain, a disease is present that requires a pill. Without a doubt, the pharmaceutical industry is dedicated to accommodating both the medical profession's calling and the layperson's unexamined desire for the quick fix—the "pill for an ill." This is a mainstay of *allopathic* medicine, the predominant medical philosophy in America, as practiced by current graduates from its medical schools. Allopathic medicine is considered the scientific version of all the healing arts.

The allopathic medical system makes and tests models of reality by what can be observed to fit certain well-defined criteria. In practice, this means an allopathic physician will focus on energy from a diagnostic perspective, measuring it with the use of electrocardiographs, electroencephalographs and electromyographs, while focusing less on how the body's energy might be used for healing.

In contrast, *alternative* medical systems are characterized by a developed body of accepted wisdom about health and its precepts that have been continuously practiced over many generations by a multitude of practitioners in many communities. To a traditional Chinese medical practitioner, for example, the focus on energy flow throughout the body and the consequence to health when it is blocked is more significant than its measurement. Simply stated, much of Western medicine holds a reductionist view of how one becomes healthy—and if an objective measurement tool for patient complaints doesn't exist, the temptation is to say a person's illness doesn't either.

The rest of the story...is functional medicine

Functional medicine is a science-based healthcare approach that assesses and treats underlying causes of illness through *individually tailored therapies* to restore health and improve function. It differs from *alternative* approaches that depend more on the integration of spiritual, ritual and empirical (gained from observation or experience) medical knowledge. And functional medicine differs from the *allopathic* approach, also known as conventional medicine, that emphasizes diagnosis of disease, followed by application of a standard treatment that is most likely to apply to a majority of patients. A *functional* medicine practitioner like Dr. Unusual is anxious to take action with a patient like BMW because he believes that prompt intervention will prevent a progression of illness that can become unbearable emotionally, spiritually, financially and physically.

He practices a type of "upstream" (studying root or underlying causes) medicine by interrupting chemical processes that could leave a person sick "downstream." Regulating blood pressure is an example. Dr. Unusual uses biochemistry, physiology, nutrition and psychosocial considerations to understand and improve physiological, emotional/cognitive and physical function. He doesn't assume that the high blood pressure a patient has is the result of the same metabolic defect in a long range of physiological actions that is universal for everyone. Similar symptoms can result from different metabolic alterations, and so addressing the "system" will be a better approach than intervention at one step along the way. If someone is already chronically ill, there are secondary preventative and therapeutic interventions that are available. By contrast, Dr. Usual will most likely suggest a pill that will effectively work to bring blood pressure down, but nothing will likely be done about the underlying causes.

The clinical impact of alterations of physiologic processes, more accurately known as "metabolic biotransformation," is astounding. Simply put, when your cells aren't communicating or are communicating an altered message, the result is reflected in almost every chronic and acute medical problem we face. While you may not yet have a "disease," if you are feeling tired, fighting your weight, are achy, have cholesterol and sugar management problems and no longer light up a room with your vim, vigor and optimism for life, you are on the way to the full-fledged development of a disease. You are limping along the road of life instead of skipping, and the destination ahead, unless dramatic changes are made, does not look like a desirable vacation resort. Unfortunately, one hundred million Americans are suffering from chronic diseases and are on that road with you.[1]

Dr. Unusual's approach

Dr. Unusual's approach is to get you to take a detour, reroute you and enable you to miss that "disease" destination. He does so by carefully analyzing what is really going on in a person's body, testing, history taking and applying well-known principles about how the body works to make the baselines clear. He then recommends interventions (specific foods, exercise, botanicals, lifestyle adjustments and traditional medicines) that affect your health. In technical terms, Dr. Unusual studies the "interconnected processes regulating the production, activity and excretion of bioactive signaling substances that promote both local change in function and 'action at a distance' through physiologic function."[2] *Translation:* He or she is going to ensure that your cells talk to each other in a way that makes you healthy.

When BMW became Dr. Unusual's patient, she thought of herself as one of many beautiful midlife women in his patient population. However, Dr. Unusual did not think of her simply as one of the crowd. He assumed instead that she was unique. This uniqueness of individual traits is a reality that must be considered when it comes to medical treatment—one size does not fit all. My husband shares the story of identical twins he had as patients who were both getting married and had come to see him to begin a birth control regimen. After some trial and error, they were placed on different products because they experienced completely different side-effect profiles. Their genes were identical, but the language spoken physiologically between genes and cells were as different as French is from English. A physician with a functional medicine mind-set will work to tailor treatment to the individual—it is "patient-centered" medicine.

Anything that assists and augments the body's natural design and the healing processes set in place by the Creator simply makes sense. The body is not a series of isolated parts but an integrated whole. The goal is to heal without creating further harm. A functional practitioner is far less apt to apply a "wait-and-see" approach to standard treatments, because he or she believes that even small imbalances can make a difference in long-term health. Suboptimal health is a factor in the development and experience of chronic illness and degenerative diseases.

For the functional doctor, the specifics of how and when to intervene are not based solely on accepted evidence as defined in a textbook or observed in a laboratory result. Treatment is not determined by an arbitrary cutoff point but through a "functional" assessment of how efficiently and effectively the body, or a specific cell, organ or system in the body, is working.

The goal in a functional approach is to find root causes and suggest interventions that work long term. A functional doctor believes that in most cases, the message your genes give the cells can be modified by the environment, diet, lifestyle, drugs and chemicals as well as many other factors. There is a consciousness that serious medical problems are "suggested" before they become full-blown. Ironically, the odds of a poor outcome can be overcome as long as we look at the minutia of the big picture. In essence, the bottom line is that we are not robots programmed by our Creator to perform physiologically (or spiritually) like everyone else in a rigid unchangeable way. Our particular unique function may require some detective work, but it is not undecipherable.

WHERE CAN I FIND MY VERY OWN
FUNCTIONAL MEDICINE DOCTOR?

If you want to pursue the possibility of treatment by a functional doctor, there are various ways to do so. There is a training center for physicians who would like to brush up on their functional medicine skills, The Institute for Functional Medicine (a nonprofit educational organization). Contacting them is a good first start for a referral in your area (www.functionalmedicine.org). Another option is to contact Great Smokies Diagnostic Laboratory (800-522-4762) since health practitioners using their services are likely familiar with a functional approach. You are also apt to find knowledgeable practitioners among doctors of osteopathy (D.O.), whose philosophy has always been to seek ways the body might heal itself. Naturopathic doctors (N.D.) are possibilities. Doctors of chiropractic (D.C.) from some schools have considerable functional training as do some nutritionists. Traditional Chinese medicine (TCM) practitioners are very functional in their approach. It has been our experience that physician assistants (P.A.), nurse practitioners (N.P.) and/or registered dieticians (R.D.) specializing in women's health are often very knowledgeable or at least open to becoming a health partner.

For most women who are not in large populated areas, chances are, like BMW, you are going to need to "make your own" physician into one with a functional "persuasion." You can do it. The first criterion is finding a practitioner who is willing to listen and work with you. If you don't feel up to that task quite yet, chapter nine will provide suggestions for you to approach your physician. In some cases, allopathic physicians will work in cooperation with an alternative practitioner who is more knowledgeable of functional assessment tools and philosophy. Until there are more allopathic physicians who are familiar with natural supplementation, testing and other procedures, this teamwork sometimes proves to be a very workable solution.

Getting the best care

Despite the numbers of Americans suffering from *chronic* diseases, allopathic medicine continues to be preoccupied with *acute* diseases (defined as having rapid onset, severe symptoms and a short course).[3] The health practitioner who listens, respects your input, considers your emotional and physical environment and metabolic balance and is sensitive to your biochemical individuality is "a keeper." Functional medicine necessitates taking a balanced approach to treatment. Such a practitioner must be willing to refer or to order potent medicines and drastic, lifesaving procedures when necessary—without allowing attention to preventative, chronic and degenerative health to be squeezed out.

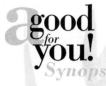

1. Do you allow yourself to question the advice given to you by a health professional?

2. Do you ask if other options exist?

3. If a doctor tells you there are no options, do you head for the door or accept what is offered?

4. Do you believe that illness and disease are inevitable?

5. In what ways is medicine a mirror image of our culture?

4

waking up the scientist within

We resolve issues and/or explore the truth with a personal bias that is ingrained within us as individuals and as creatures of our culture. Sometimes scientists fall short of acknowledging their bias. The scientific method was developed in part to remove personal bias from the experimental process. However, being the emotional creatures we are, even scientists are inevitably influenced by their personal life experience such as the need for acceptance, financial pursuit or response to personal or family illnesses to which they have been exposed. This faulty predisposition influences research interests as well as interpretation of results. Pure science does not exist; it never did, and it never will.

That does not give us an excuse to zone out and not think scientifically about a doctor's recommendation. There is a tendency for us to trust the specialist and not think critically about what is being offered. Admittedly, there is much to learn, and it is common to feel deficient when we can't even pronounce the medical jargon. But there is a great difference between understanding it all and thinking critically.

THE INNER SCIENTIST

Our inner scientist is capable of systematically assessing what is being presented and coming to a conclusion in a professional setting—in other words, thinking critically—about whether or not the specialist knows what he or she is doing. Yes, it requires some background about how the body works, and some effort must be expended. You are reading this book for that reason.

Thinking like a scientist is like falling off a log

In case you aren't convinced that an inner scientist exists at the core of your being, let's look at two quite ordinary examples of scientific decision making. We will start with Mary Jane. She is a new mother, enamored with her six-week-old daughter. She is at peace with her decision to stay home with baby Anna and has given little thought to her former life as a high-powered executive. The same diligence, care and minute observation she previously focused on financial printouts and year-end reports are now reserved entirely for Anna. Even when the baby is sleeping, Mary Jane watches every twitch and bubble, speculating about what sweet thoughts are flowing through those baby synapses and neurons. Her powers of observation are such that she increasingly anticipates Anna's needs even before a cry makes them unavoidable.

something to think about

Pure science does not exist; it never did, and it never will.

Last Saturday, Mary Jane's careful interpretation of her child's behavior led her to the conclusion that something was wrong. Anna was not herself; she seemed stiff and listless. She was running a fever. A call to her pediatric group assured her that it was probably nothing serious; she was instructed in ways to reduce the fever. Unconvinced, several hours later, the subtle but disturbing difference in Anna's behavior prompted Mary Jane to take her to the emergency room, where she was diagnosed with meningitis.

A second example involves Celeste, a bright and happy three-year-old. On a trip with her mother to the grocery store, she decided she wanted a box of cereal her mother did not want her to have. At first she asked nicely, but getting no response, she began to whine. Her mother ignored her. She proceeded to cry softly and as pitifully as possible, a maneuver that always worked with her father. Her mother responded with irritation. Celeste waited until an audience gathered in the aisle and then began to wail at the top of her lungs. Embarrassed, her mother quickly placed the cereal into the basket and moved on.

Mary Jane and Celeste were acting like scientists. They were using the same "scientific method" you may vaguely remember discussed in high school science class. They defined a problem, analyzed the variables, came up with a hypothesis, tested their theory, observed the results, decided whether the problem was solved and had on reserve another hypothesis to put into play should the first prove, experientially, not to work.

The entire scientific process was not beyond the scope of a three-year-old. Celeste wanted her cereal (the problem). She had to convince her mother to buy it. She tried asking nicely because her experience with her mother had been that she was a reasonable person who often got her what she wanted (analyzed the variables). But this time, Mom was tough. So Celeste tried to evoke pity; it backfired. Having attempted and failed at more moderate methods, she used her "big gun"–humiliation. It worked, and Celeste added the last line to her scientific procedure (the conclusion). It was, of course, that throwing tantrums in front of people gets you what you want.

In our first example, Mary Jane gathered information on both a physical and emotional level just like Celeste, but it was of no value until it was applied. Mary Jane's observation that her child was not acting in her usual way provided the impetus to take appropriate action to decipher the mystery of what was going on. Thinking like a scientist is, for most, a nonconscious act. Every time you astutely observe something, you are doing what scientists do. A scientist thinks critically about his or her observations and then applies the information. Even scientists sometimes miss this point, failing to make the distinction between discovery and application. Conclusions derived from scientific observations and discoveries are not an end in themselves, no matter how grand. It is their appropriate use or application that counts.

But an additional caution is in order. The applications made from scientific observations are inherently influenced by the bias of the observer. Mary Jane suspected her child was ill. Her action was to seek the opinion of a medical authority. Had she been a Christian Scientist, she may have contacted her clergy leaders. If she lived in the Amazon, her first stop might have been a shaman.

Keeping the arguments logical

What is relevant in thinking like a scientist is the ability to identify whether an argument is logical or not. If the assumptions under which recommendations are made are flawed, then the suggestions are flawed. Look at what happened with hormone replacement therapy, for example. The conventional wisdom that women need medicinal hormones at menopause implies a number of notions about aging. Assumptions such as:

> *If* menopause is a disease, *then* all women who stop making estrogen in the amounts they did as young women are going to become ill very soon after they stop menstruating and will get sick and die at a relatively young age as compared to men.

Is this true? No. Women do not die in association with the fact that they are no longer able to reproduce. Closer scrutiny, a reality check, if you will, reveals:

1. Women on average outlive men.

2. Hormones don't disappear completely; they decline gradually and continue to support bone, heart health and other vital functions.

3. There appears to be an adaptive advantage to socializing humans when several generations are involved. Mature adults possessing wisdom and insight most profoundly influence the young when the business and distraction of childbearing and child rearing come to an end. So, declining hormones are part of aging, but not a death sentence.

If menopause were truly a disease, then needing a pill to fix it is a logical conclusion. A "pill-for-an-ill" mentality permeates our daily life, as we have mentioned, expressing itself when we grab an aspirin rather than taking a walk or scrutinizing superficially truths we would rather avoid. In the scientific community, this "quick-fix" mentality directs research to focus on the latest, greatest, fastest magical-make-it-right medication. But popping a pill at midlife won't result in healthy aging, a healthy menopause and a balanced life. It makes no difference how dramatic the outcomes in the short run, ultimately all pills are a temporary fix *if they are not addressing the underlying cause of the problem at hand.* Whether you use herbs, vitamins, minerals, biofeedback, acupuncture, massage, chiropractic, osteopathy, Ayurveda or Chinese medicine, *if you treat the symptom and not the cause,* the outcome will always be disappointing.

Your body is a divine complexity; a philosophy of simplistic reductionism does not make it otherwise. The bias of *Good for You!* is clearly to require you to reflect on a complete and very big picture and to think critically while you are at it. There is no suggestion that you forgo any medication from this time forth—just that you accept the reality that "there is no free lunch." We intend to walk you through the process of "thinking big" by providing examples of a functional and multidisciplinary model for health.

Sharing the same boat

Our point is that specialists are not the only ones to have the right vocabulary of a critically thinking mind. You are perfectly capable of making well-informed medical decisions, especially when you have examined your own personal assumptions. However, the tendency, as we have stated, is to abdicate responsibility and leave the application of scientific observations to medical scientists. As you have seen, this may not be the wisest thing to do in matters of your health. Scientists practice good and sloppy science and exhibit rational and irrational thinking. Laypeople do the same. The use of critical thinking can be selective.

So what does all this have to do with your health, menopause and hormones? Let's make sure you are clear. Thinking like a scientist means you have a systematic way of evaluating assumptions and testing ideas or solving problems. A set of steps exists. You use them unconsciously all the time. You can also choose to use them *consciously* when dealing with complex matters of your health. We are simply reminding and encouraging you to do what you already know how to do. And we are giving you multifaceted information with which to do it.

With the current breakdown in what has heretofore been considered acceptable treatment for menopause and beyond, there is every reason to start doing what you have been avoiding–making critical thinking choices regarding your health. Our expectations for the medical community have been too high. Consider, for example, the possibility that our increased education and ability to access information has lulled us into depending too much on scientific knowledge and not enough on thoughtful application of that knowledge.

Good for You! was written to provide information that is good for you and to remind you to use critical thinking to assess your health issues– testing and applying what is appropriate for your situation. The process is like coming to a conclusion after sitting on a jury. Every citizen, with few exceptions, is considered capable of judging guilt or innocence, evaluating extenuating circumstances and sometimes determining life or death sentences. A jurist is given facts and asked to see both sides. A decision must be made as to whom to believe and whether experts are credible. Personal assumptions must be scrutinized to keep the matter in its proper perspective.

something
to think about

If you, as a woman, are capable of critical thinking, then you will be able to make healthy, life-affirming decisions.

This process is no different from what is being asked of you when deciding what to do about hormone health, natural supplements and products to delay aging. Just like the jurist, you make a good decision you can live with, having heard the whole story.

You see, we have an assumption about you. It is:

> If you, as a woman, are capable of critical thinking, *then* you will be able to make healthy, life-affirming decisions.

Meaning, you will take sometimes complex materials, test and determine a plan that results in your personal optimal wellness with a risk level that is suitable and appropriate for you. If your plan works, that's great. If it does not, you will go back to the drawing board to review where you went astray and where you will go next—like a scientist.

GOOD FOR YOU! THINKING

Functional medicine defines disease as "dysfunctional intercellular communication." As you consider the way you have lived and how you make decisions, and examine the choices made regarding your health, you will become increasingly sensitive to how your biochemical communication is going. You will become aware of what may be blocking clear communication within and between cells and systems—and between yourself and medical personnel.

Decisions about hormone health, reducing health risks and eliminating or minimizing symptoms are approached in many different ways. The path to doing so most effectively is to first address your mind. How do you think about your health? How do you process information about the way your body works? Take the time you need to figure it out—because it will influence the choices you make. In the end, *good medicine* must be defined by *you*.

One of the reasons for recalling and analyzing your personal story is its value in helping you to become aware of how you use (or misuse) this natural ability to observe, reason and sort things out. The prototype with which you have habitually approached your health will likely be what you will draw upon in the future. But, barring earlier medical crises, the stakes are likely to be higher; therefore, some cleaning up of one's particular scientific method is in order. It can give you confidence in your capacity to make sound decisions, even conflicting medical ones.

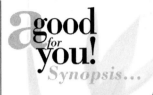

Synopsis...

Our goal is to make the unconscious conscious. Before reading further, can you identify at least three specific beliefs that underlie your health choices? If not, complete the following questions:

1. Anything related to my health scares (concerns) me because in the past _____. As a result, I do [what] _____ and feel [what]

_____.

2. I am indifferent (positive) about my health because _____. As a result, I do [what] _____ and feel [what] _____.

5

avoiding knee-jerk reactions

In chapter two, Lyra and I shared our stories and how assumptions about life, medicine and, most of all, our fears influenced the decisions we made about our personal path to health. We have asked for the same introspection from you. Undoubtedly, a lucky few have discovered that you escaped forming the emotional or physical biases that the rest of us have acted upon. *Good for you!*

The majority of you have thought about your story and perhaps realized for the first time that your assumptions and life experiences have influenced both your willingness to take health risks as well as how conscientiously you pursued your personal optimal health. You may have exposed the tendency to put thinking about it on hold and uncovered that you rely almost entirely on the suggestions of a physician. You do not need to be clairvoyant to know that at least some choices made when you didn't think like a scientist have resulted in outcomes you didn't expect. It is also possible that the choices looked right in the short term but, from a long-term perspective, are not what you anticipated. Whatever your story, you own it, and you alone can determine how else you might like to write it.

You are not alone. What follows are scenarios that we have been hearing of late. They are what might be called "knee-jerk reactions" because they are quick decisions, made as a result of the Women's Health Initiative's (WHI) recommendations that women and their doctors rethink the use of HRT. They are not decisions based on critical thinking; they are "shooting from the hip." There are commonalities: The outcome is indeterminate, and the spotlight is on the quick fix. There is an emphasis on chasing symptoms to get relief. Individual risks tend to be overlooked or ignored. You may recognize yourself. Have you already given a knee-jerk reaction a whirl, or are you thinking about it? Are you willing to do something else? Can you use your critical-thinking skills and approach what you will do next like a scientist?

COMMON KNEE-JERK REACTIONS

Carefully consider the following scenarios and determine your approach to what we are characterizing as common knee-jerk reactions:

If *pharmaceutical* hormones (HRT) are the problem, then *natural* hormones (nature-identical hormones) are the answer.

When the results of the Women's Health Initiative (WHI) were announced, Sue Ellen knew exactly what she wanted to do. Like most of her friends, she had been using traditional hormone replacement—in her case for thirteen years, the last five on Prempro, one of the drugs specifically named in the WHI report. She occasionally considered discontinuing its use, but each time she attempted to quit taking hormones, her increased hot flashes convinced her she couldn't live without them. Nevertheless, she worried about their safety, especially after discussions with her friends or following a news report that raised some new hormonal concern. Truthfully though, most of the time she gave little thought to her regimen—at least until the summer of 2002 when she could ignore it no longer.

Currently, Sue Ellen has no serious health concerns of which she is aware. At fifty-eight years of age, she uses hormones for relief of her hot flashes as well as complaints of general dryness and vaginal lubrication. A stint of painful intercourse severe enough to impact her sexual relations with her husband was the motivation for beginning weekly use of vaginal estrogen cream.

Ideally, before a new plan is adopted, Sue Ellen should make a full evaluation of her health, with baseline tests and closer scrutiny of her family history. Instead, her focus revolves around her unease about conventional hormone therapy. In her mind, maintaining good health is defined by discontinuing pharmaceutical hormones and beginning "nature-identical" ones. *I will change to nature-identical hormones because they come from plants and are similar to the ones my body makes*, she reasons.

Were you *wondering*? Pharmaceutically produced estrogen can be derived from pregnant horse's urine, the Mexican yam or soy; it can also be synthesized chemically. Pharmaceutical progestogen is chiefly from soy or the Mexican yam or can be synthesized chemically as progestin. Nature-identical estrogen or progesterone is made from Mexican yam or soy, generally in smaller laboratories or in compounding pharmacies, and from a molecular standpoint, it looks like hormones made by the body.

Is she doing the right thing? How logical is her thinking? Is she thinking critically? Essentially she is saying, "I need hormones, so I will take ones that I feel are safest." She does not question whether or not it is reasonable to add hormones to a system that is requiring far less of them to function. She ignores the risk that there is no well-documented scientific data to support her new choice—just as there was no definitive research for mare's urine (Premarin).

After an initial adjustment with nature-identical estrogen and progesterone from a compounding pharmacy, Sue Ellen is more convinced than ever that she has made the best decision for her health. She feels good on her new regimen, her hot flashes are manageable, and she has merely had to substitute a natural estrogen product to take care of her vaginal dryness. Life goes on without skipping much of a beat.

She has ignored other possible choices that lie in lifestyle practices and use of natural botanical products that keep menopausal/aging symptoms at bay while contributing to optimal health—without risk. And she has given no thought to her very real cardiovascular risk and other considerations of healthy aging. With both parents suffering from heart disease, the fact that she is overweight and has high blood pressure is significant and dangerously overlooked. She may even be doing harm—at this point there is no assurance that long-term use of nature-identical hormones won't increase her risk of breast cancer and blood clots or worsen her cardiovascular issues, just as her previous hormone use did.

Sue Ellen does not consider, either, that her hot flashes may be related to her high-stress life or perhaps thyroid imbalance, rather than menopause. Or perhaps they are due to her poor adrenal gland function and its inability to make up for hormones no longer produced in her ovaries. The truth is, Sue Ellen's attention should be directed to the larger picture of improving her nutrition, upgrading her vitamins and increasing her exercise. Such lifestyle interventions will do more for her (and be safer and far less expensive) than the hope she puts in a quick fix of "natural" hormones her body no longer needs. Her story is typical of what happens when an unconscious bias overrides a comprehensive evaluation of one's health.

If I *feel* better on HRT, then I can stay on it, as long as I cut down on how much I use.

Lorraine is fifty, but she doesn't look it. She has never felt better emotionally or physically. For the first time in her life she is able to organize her life as she desires. A lifelong gardener, she now has the time to be involved in organizations of like-minded individuals. While she is still working part time, her life feels balanced, and she wants nothing to disrupt it. The WHI study results concern her, but she views any health risk to her personally as unlikely.

Lorraine has selected the fact that she feels good as the pertinent information on which she focuses. She has decided that HRT is at least partially responsible for her sense of well-being, and as a bonus, there are few wrinkles on her face. Finding a way to hang on to HRT and at the same time reduce its risk is important to her. Without consulting her gynecologist, she makes the decision to take her hormone pills every other day. What are her consequences? Is she thinking critically?

Lorraine may find out that she feels fine on this regimen. However, her white ethnicity, a stint of bulimia in her teens and a small frame in combination with the lowered dose of estrogen increases her inherent risk for osteoporosis. HRT's bone-protecting effects are dependent on an adequate dose; the arbitrary reduction of her dosage may not meet that requirement. Given her family history of hip fractures and the fact that the alcohol she consumes can also be adding to her risk, she truly cannot know where she stands unless she makes the effort to test her bone strength. If a DXA test reveals her bones are strong, her regimen, while it might not prevent bone loss, may be acceptable—assuming she also feels that any risk she assumes is worth the quality of life she is experiencing. If, however, her bone test reveals she is osteoporotic or close to it, adequate dosage level is imperative.

Lorraine's failure to examine the bias (feeling good) that drives her to continue a capricious dosage of HRT subjects her to the risk that it may not be doing the good it is capable of, which may be increasing the risk of serious health problems down the road. Worst of all, it keeps her from examining her true baseline health and may put her at risk for a preventable disease.

If I don't want to or no longer feel I can use hormone therapy, then I will protect myself by buying all natural products from the health food store.

A related assumption might be, if I am menopausal, then I have to *do something*.

Beth is a forty-eight-year-old hairdresser whose last period was three months ago. She has read many of the alternative books on menopause and, of course, is privy to plenty of advice from her customers. She thinks a lot about exercising, but she finds that after leaving the shop she is simply too exhausted. She has cut down on her smoking, limiting herself to two cigarettes a day.

She hasn't had a physical exam for five years. At that time, her doctor gave her a prescription for HRT, which she filled and took for three months before deciding to quit because of worry about its safety and the realization that she didn't feel good on it. She continued to fill her prescription for Paxil, which has been renewed over the phone at her request. Despite infrequent visits to her physician, she is somewhat of a hypochondriac and worries about coming down with a serious disease—often ones she hears about in the media. Three or four times a year she visits a chiropractor who treats an ongoing back problem and advises her on the use of natural products.

Beth has had to clear a shelf in her kitchen to hold all the natural products she has purchased. She is right to be concerned about staying healthy as she ages, but her shotgun approach means that much of what she does is wasted. The data she is selecting to pay attention to is, *I am at risk,* rather than, *What is really going on in my body?* Instead of going to her doctor for laboratory tests that can give her black-and-white evidence as to the true state of her health and reviewing family history, her personal lifestyle and medical history, she is casting a wide net in hopes of covering anything that might be wrong.

Her approach of *doing something* is expensive monetarily and risky from a health standpoint. Her habit of becoming her own pharmacist means that the vitamin and mineral ratios of the body that are important for proper metabolism can become skewed. Depletion factors and interactions are likely. To give herself an emotional "edge," for example, she began taking St. John's wort with her Paxil, a questionable and potentially dangerous combination that might lead to overdose.

To be a wise consumer in a conventional medical world unfamiliar with supplements and plants, she should be careful about mixing concentrated herbal products with pharmaceutical prescriptions or even commonly used over-the-counter medications like aspirin, ibuprofen and so on. Most importantly, she may very well be mistreating or ignoring a serious undisclosed health condition. With her *more-is-better-as-long-as-it-is-natural* approach, there is no way of knowing for sure.

---

onsider *this...* Informing a new physician of everything you are taking is critical to avoid drug interactions. In 1997, sixty million Americans claimed to use herbs, and 70 percent of them did not reveal herb use to their medical doctor or pharmacist.[1]

Whatever Beth takes should be justifiable, preferably by a demonstrated need. Her prescriptions were not written for continual use and need to be reevaluated within a reasonable time. Beth's interest in staying healthy is commendable. Her belief that almost anything you take will help is not. Especially disturbing is her focus on "pill popping" as a substitute for other healthful actions like stopping smoking, exercising and the necessity for special interventions, due to the fact she works in a toxic environment.

Beth believes she alone is able to stay on top of her health, but she needs a health coach—conventional or alternative. *The doctors say herbs are dangerous, but they are the same ones who said hormones weren't,* she tells herself. Whatever Beth's true medical issues, there is no reason to panic and plenty of reason to take the time to gather a complete health history before deciding on a plan of action. After all, we need to remember that neither getting old nor menopause is a disease.

If hormones cause serious health problems, then I should never take them.

Doreen is a natural beauty in many ways. She is athletic and in much better shape than most forty-five-year-old women. When she was in college, she was a long-distance runner, unusual for women of that era. She did not start her periods until she was sixteen, and although she has two children, she had a very difficult time conceiving. She takes a multivitamin she purchases at the grocery store and uses TUMS as her calcium source. She has noticed that she has more wrinkles than her peers, a fact she attributes to the time she has spent in outdoor activities, although she has always tried to be diligent about the use of sunscreen.

Two years ago, Doreen adamantly refused her doctor's suggestion to begin HRT for general prevention and hot flash relief and feels vindicated for that decision by the recent WHI report. She assumes that if she continues her healthy lifestyle, she will not need medication. Her assumption appears sound, but it has blinded her to the possibility that good health is a combination of lifestyle and genetic propensity. In reality, Doreen is someone who would benefit from hormone therapy. Her low body fat, the result of years of intensive exercise, the late onset of periods, difficulty conceiving and even her wrinkles are suggestive of ovarian dysfunction.

onsider *this...* A DXA (Dual-energy X-ray Absorptiometry) is a noninvasive test that measures how strong your bones are and your risk of fracture. A simple urinalysis that measures N-telopeptide or pyridinium crosslinks/deoxypyridinoline can track the success of your new strategy in the short term. Elevated levels indicate bone breakdown; normal levels suggest bone stability and a successful intervention.

It was a serendipitous happening for Doreen that led to an Achilles-heel bone density test at a health fair, which revealed she might be osteoporotic. A follow-up with a DXA confirmed full-fledged osteoporosis. At first Doreen's knee-jerk reaction adamantly refused her physician's assessment that she must consider hormone therapy or selective estrogen receptor modulators (SERMs). Further reading helped her realize that while lifestyle adjustments would be critical in preventing further bone loss, her imminent risk of debilitating pain and broken bones necessitated action. Fortunately, she put her critical thinking skills to work.

Doreen immediately shifted to a more effective calcium product and increased the potency of her vitamins as a result of sharing her story with a knowledgeable natural-medicine-oriented nutritionist. Acknowledging that she could not escape some risk if she was to control further bone loss, she educated herself on her options. She decided on a regimen of a soy-based estrogen with nature-identical progesterone added the last two weeks of the month—the combination that appears to have the least potential risk. She will continue to monitor new information as it is released and as new treatments unfold.

She did not take her physician's suggestion to use one of the new SERMs, preferring instead to stick with a drug that had been around longer and whose risks and benefits were more specifically known. Her selection was made easier by the fact that her family history did not include breast cancer or heart disease, and it was based partly on her own good cardio-vascular health.

Doreen could have continued to refuse hormones. To do so would mean accepting the increased risk of a spinal or hip fracture. However, the value she placed on being active made it important to her to stop any further bone loss and to build as much bone as possible.

If hormones cause breast cancer, then I have cancer because I took them.

Pat just celebrated her sixty-third birthday. There were times this last year when she didn't know if she would make it or if she wanted to. Six months of chemotherapy followed by radiation kept her nauseated and weak throughout most of the year. While her days have been spent focusing on the "tyranny of the urgent"–getting to the next doctor's appointment or managing her prescriptions–free moments found her berating herself for not taking seriously the risk of breast cancer as a result of estrogen use.

She gladly filled her first HRT prescription fifteen years ago. HRT controlled her hot flashes and enabled her to breeze through perimenopause and menopause with minimal difficulty. But had she known what she was to face down the road, she never would have been so glib or unquestioning.

> **C**onsider *this*... Out of every fifty-six American women, twenty-eight can expect to die from heart disease, eight will develop osteoporosis, and seven will develop breast cancer.[2]

Of all the observations Pat could make about why she developed breast cancer, she selected *hormone therapy* as her focus. It was known to increase the chance of breast cancer; therefore, she concluded, it was responsible. While there is no way to prove the definitive factor leading to any disease, it is clear that whatever role HRT played, it was only a player, not the orchestrator. There were other players involved–like having only one child at a late age, the two glasses of wine she consumed daily, her high-fat diet, a late menopause, her disdain for vegetables and the extra pounds she was carrying.

We do not know whether Pat would have developed breast cancer if she had attended to all these risk factors. We do know that despite our best efforts, people do suffer serious illness. No one intervention will make or break the process. Self-blame is not healing, but moving on can be.

AND WHAT ABOUT YOU?

This is a critical time. It is tempting to grab at the nearest straw, if for no other reason than to still the anxiety. Have you acknowledged how terrified you are upon learning that what to do to keep healthy is not going to be found in a pill? Maybe your fear feels like anger at the medical community in which you put your trust. Perhaps you are resigned to thinking that it is all a speculation and you have no other choices. Maybe fear has boomeranged, and you feel guilty for having bought the HRT myth. Or perhaps it is your resentment that you need it and feel better with it and it is going to be taken away.

There is no doubt that all people have a personal myopia about the choice of data on which we make our assumptions and from which we take action. We are asking you to be mindful of the power of these faulty assumptions.

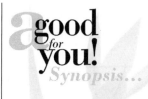

1. Are you aware of any assumptions you have made about your health?
2. Is your focus on your health or on a solution somewhat myopic?
3. Do you find yourself chasing symptoms?
4. Do you fail to find the time to see your practitioner for a checkup?
5. Who controls your body?

6

when estrogen does what it does best

Lucy is only thirty-three years old, but her periods have become lighter each month. She is embarrassed to admit it, but she has begun experiencing hot flashes during stressful times at work. She called her doctor, who said she was too young to be menopausal. A sense of unwellness permeates her spirit.

Janene is forty-eight years old. At her annual checkup her doctor announced her hormone levels indicated she was perimenopausal. She was shocked, since she had been feeling the same as always.

It is her friend, Shirley, by contrast, who has become a walking menopause textbook. It seems to Janene that Shirley suffers from every symptom ever associated with menopause. Janene worries that one day she will wake up and find herself equally miserable.

It is notable that while each of these women is experiencing a real life-changing occurrence, the pattern of the change does not fit a typical menopause mold. That is because there isn't one.

MENOPAUSE DEFINED

Menopause is a communal experience shared with all women of every culture. While individual women may marry or not, give birth or not and only randomly find themselves on the same twenty-eight-day menstrual cycles with women around the world, if they live long enough, they will all go through menopause. Menopause signals the end of the body's ability to reproduce—it is a most natural event. With it comes a shift in a woman's life focus and the nonescapable reality that her days are to be lived in a new way.

For some women that means an opportunity to share the wisdom learned from life experience, while others find they are finally able to attend to things passed over during the years when life had more demands. Still others relish the new rhythm they previously had only dreamed their life would have. Sadly, many women's lives do not unfold so beautifully. Caretaking responsibilities can be extended to include aging parents or grandchildren, a role that has grown appropriately tiresome. Some, like Shirley, find the physical transition of menopause to be severe and uncomfortable.

The average age for menopause is fifty-one years. A woman is officially postmenopausal when periods have stopped for twelve months. The transition to the point where there are no more viable eggs in the ovaries does not happen overnight, even if a woman's change appears as simple as never having another period. Women in their thirties and forties may sense subtle changes that can be considered "premenopausal." Symptoms and signs become more evident five years before periods actually stop. This is called "perimenopause," and for many women, it is the most problematic time of their "change of life."

Lucy, at thirty-three, does not fit the norm; however, she is not unusual. It is possible to become menopausal at an early age due to genetic factors or medical complications such as hysterectomy or chemotherapy. Without laboratory testing for confirmation, a woman should never be dismissed as "too young" to experience menopause. Another cause of an earlier menopause is smoking.

Janene is fortunate to have few symptoms of menopause. Her genetic makeup and the general condition of her health are most likely the salient factors. Janene has always eaten well, taken nutritional supplements and been a stickler for a daily exercise regimen. There is no doubt that the healthier a woman is when she enters menopause, the fewer her problems—remember Lyra.

It follows that if interventions are used to control symptoms, they can be less powerful. The difficult experience of Janene's friend, Shirley, may reflect her genes, lifestyle factors, how stress is handled or illnesses she has or has had in the past. Even her expectations and the meaning she gives this life conversion could play a part in making her transition difficult.

MENOPAUSE COMES WITH BAGGAGE

An unfortunate thing about menopause is that it occurs at the same time a woman's body may begin to manifest symptoms of degenerative disease.

Such illnesses are often chronic and tend to increase in intensity with age. While a woman may hear about a problem for the first time during peri-menopause, the disease process has been insidiously taking place for years. A lifetime of stealth work by disease is merely accelerated by the drop in estrogen at menopause.

You do not become osteoporotic, for example, because you are menopausal; the reduction in estrogen at midlife is not the mitigating factor in its development. For example, seeds for osteoporosis may be planted when, as a teenage girl, the decision was made to reduce calories by avoiding cheese and milk. That choice resulted in calcium being in short supply and not amply available during this crucial bone-building time.

Should the same woman quit doing weight-bearing exercise after college, at thirty-five when bone buildup is finished and bone loss normally begins, her increased loss at midlife becomes significant. By contrast, a woman who enters menopause with strong bones can withstand the five-year increased loss that occurs when periods stop.

You may also have concurrent health concerns, both large and small, that can conveniently be labeled "menopausal" but, in truth, have little to do with "change-of-life" issues. It is important to make the distinction because what you decide to do for menopause, as opposed to treatment modalities for diseases, can be very different. Making a distinction between a symptom of menopause and a symptom of disease is not always as obvious as one might think.

onsider *this…* The most prominent hormonal change of menopause is a dramatic reduction in circulating estradiol levels (10–20 pg/ml). The symptom most clearly linked to menopause is hot flash. The most prominent complaint associated with menopause is joint ache and pain.[1]

MENOPAUSE ASSUMPTIONS

The faulty perception remains that menopause either is a disease or causes disease. But think about it. All older women go through menopause; most do not develop debilitating diseases following their final period. Women who aren't menopausal can have heart attacks and become osteoporotic. The point is that chronic health risk is *coincidental* with menopause, not *causative*.

What is *true* is that how a woman has lived her life will affect how she experiences menopause and her propensity for developing a disease. Most women are comfortable with the concept that procreation is not the sole reason for their existence. Ordinary and extraordinary women frequently experience renewed vitality and a redirected creative force after menopause.

Since menopause is not a disease, taking medicine to get over it is unnecessary. Estrogen and progesterone define physical femininity and are instrumental for reproduction; they are no longer needed at high levels when that is no longer the body's agenda. The body wisely turns down reproductive hormonal function at a certain age, but continues producing the same hormones at levels below those that maintain fertility. There are many redundant systems—hormones are produced in the skin, brain and fat from other precursor hormones when the ovaries are no longer the chief source.

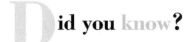 **id you know?** Typical clinical changes of menopause include menstrual irregularities four years before, hormonal changes eight years before and a decline in fertility up to ten years before menses cease.[2]

A woman's perfect design was never to accommodate proliferative levels of hormones every day, every hour. Estrogen and progesterone wax and wane throughout the month, even releasing in a pulsing fashion throughout the day. This natural rhythm spares hormone-sensitive tissue like the breast, uterus, vagina and endometrium from continued exposure to these highly stimulating agents. Where is the wisdom in supplementing hormones outside the normal range of our biological clock? How does the body cope? What systems are responsible for clearing unwanted hormones?

EXACTLY WHAT DOES ESTROGEN DO?

I can hear some of you moaning all the way to my office. "Why must I know what estrogen does?" you ask. "Just tell me what to take instead." And I say to you, "Ahh, if it were only that simple!" I'm afraid there is no avoiding exercising some synapses and building some neurons in your brain. I promise, learning about estrogen (and more) will be *good for you!*

Hormone replacement therapy (HRT) may have become dirty words, but, believe me, you do not want to live without hormones. Considering that hormones were not even discovered until the early 1900s, it should be no surprise that we are only now uncovering information about their good and bad effects. Basically, hormones are signaling messengers involved in almost every chemical process in our body. They influence growth, metabolism, strength, endurance and vitality. Hormones even control other hormones. Keeping them in a balance appropriate for one's age and stage in life increases your chance of good health and well-being. Helping you learn how to do that is one of the goals of this book.

Here again, we must look at this material from a functional model perspective, determining how your systems communicate. Why? Because if we don't, we are apt to take the simple way out—and you won't build all those new synapses. You see, it would be nice if we could consider menopause a function of declining estrogen and progesterone. But the reality is, we can only understand estrogen/progesterone and its relationship to menopause if we understand the interplay of several hormones.

Annoying midlife symptoms, which for many last far beyond menopause, reflect the complex interactions of multiple systems: the hypothalamus-pituitary-ovarian axis. They are the result of hormonal communication or miscommunication. Ultimately, it's all about clear communication between cells and systems that operate on delicate feedback loops. When you factor in "organ reserve" (the little extra you have stashed away for a rainy day) that dwindles over time due to genetics and environment, the clinical picture becomes infinitely complex. In a nutshell, more than estrogen is involved; the real deal involves hormonal cross-talk.

While we speak most often about *estrogen,* in reality there are three versions of varying potency: estradiol (E2), estrone (E1) and estriol (E3). E2 is the strongest and E3 is the weakest. All three versions of estrogen, if given in strong enough doses, can act like estradiol. Consider this fact when you decide that adding hormones will be safe as long as you stick to the "weakest" version, estriol.

When estrogen and progesterone leave corporate headquarters

When estrogen is prescribed by a physician and taken as a pill, lozenge or through the skin, it is called *exogenous*—from an outside source. You can also take in exogenous estrogen through the foods you eat and from chemicals to which you are exposed, like pesticides that mimic hormones.

The estrogen you make in your body is known as *endogenous*. In perimenopause, before menstrual cycles stop completely, the depletion of egg follicles in the ovary results in a steady decline of estrogen, although its measurement in the bloodstream can vary considerably. After menopause, the main source of estrogen is from conversion of a precursor hormone called androstenedione that is made in the adrenal gland. Obviously, entering menopause with healthy adrenals is important. By the time a woman is well into her postmenopausal years, most estradiol is derived from testosterone, but the predominant estrogen in circulation remains estrone.

Breast tissue, the brain, bone, coronary arteries and the lining of the uterus are prime sites for final conversion stages of estrogen. Whether this is good or bad depends on many things. A healthy wallop of estrogen converted in the bone is beneficial, while in other tissues, like the breast, it can prove harmful. The level of estrogen production in various areas of the body increases with age and weight. Generally, a person with more fat cells is going to produce more estrogen. Because a woman's need for estrogen continues, the Divine Architect of the body made sure estrogen production would carry on.

Estrogen's taxi service

Once estrogen is produced it must move around the body in order to enter target-tissue cells and induce biological activity. Only about 2–3 percent is free to roam about on its own. The majority of the free estrogen combines with "sex-hormone-binding globulin" (SHBG). SHBG is somewhat like a taxi, and if something alters the amount available, it will influence the quantity of free estrogen—just as pulling taxis out of service leaves people to get around on their own. This is important because when estrogen is riding in the taxi, it is unable to do its work.

How estrogen gets a second chance

Once estrogen has made its way around the body and prompted a cell to respond to the message it carries, it ultimately makes its way to the liver where it is broken down and bound to bile acids, excreted into the gastrointestinal tract and finally eliminated as feces or through the kidneys as urine. If, however, a woman's bowel is inhabited by the wrong kind of bacteria, estrogen can be reabsorbed and passed through the liver again to begin another trek, with another opportunity to influence cellular metabolism. And if your intestinal tract is poorly functioning, estrogen may be reabsorbed at a level your body cannot manage, or it could allow an overabundance back into your system.

Production of "good-girl" and "bad-girl" estrogen

When it comes to staying healthy or getting sick, research tells us that the way estrogen is broken down is more important than any gene you may be lucky or unlucky enough to have inherited. These breakdown products have significant biologic effects that in some cases may influence the safety and efficacy of the estrogen your body makes or that you add through what you eat or take medicinally. We will talk more about how good estrogen can go bad and how you can keep that from happening in the next chapter.

Were you *wondering*? When estrogen is a good girl, it...

- Combats dryness generally
- Lowers bad LDL cholesterol
- Has antioxidant effects
- Reduces risk of colon cancer
- Improves skin; reduces wrinkling
- Is neuro-protective of brain
- Reduces glaucoma
- Influences mood
- Helps prevent urinary urgency and leakage
- Helps maintain vaginal health and comfort
- Maintains bone density

The importance of the right parking place

How estrogen affects a cell and sets into motion a series of good or bad events is determined by which form of estrogen it is, how the liver breaks it down, a woman's genes, cell chemistry and the particular receptor to which it binds. A receptor is like a parking place. It is the literal spot on the cell where estrogen attaches. What happens when it parks is determined by proteins, pathways and processes by which receptors interact. There are two types, alpha and beta, and several subtypes of each. This explains why the body can respond to the same hormone differently—the parking spots are different. For instance, when estradiol binds to the *alpha* receptor, it tells the cell to begin certain chemical reactions; when it binds to the beta receptor, the message activated is exactly the opposite of what it set in motion with the alpha receptor.[3] (Note: The alpha receptor was discovered in 1986, the beta in 1996. These dates remind us how very new estrogen science happens to be.)

The time estrogen spends in its preferred parking place determines the biologic activity and, with respect to hormone therapy, the potency of the prescribed hormone. Estrogen receptors will bind with other than free estrogen. Many toxins and plant cells can park at a receptor with varying affinity and action. This is why so much of the current pharmaceutical research on hormones is geared toward the development of selective estrogen receptor modulators—SERMs—designer drugs that can activate some but not all target cells.

In some cases when these designer drugs are used, estrogen action is blocked; in others, it is stimulated. For example, the SERM raloxifene stimulates bone growth through its action at the estrogen receptor, but it does not have a proliferative effect on breast and endometrial tissue. However, in the brain, it acts in an antiestrogen way, making it more difficult for blood vessels to constrict and dilate appropriately, which may cause a woman taking raloxifene to experience increased hot flashes.

onsider *this…* Accumulating evidence indicates it is not estrogen—as either estradiol or estrone—but estrogen metabolites that may be contributing to the health risks associated with estrogen during menstruation, at the menopause or with hormone replacement therapy.

—JEFFREY S. BLAND, PH.D.[4]

Plant-derived isoflavones and lignans and their metabolites can be considered *natural* SERMs. Although often referred to as "phytoestrogens," their actions on the cell are not that of an estrogen. They function in an agonist/antagonist fashion, or as an "adaptogen." Adaptogens have a balancing effect on the body, working in whatever direction is needed, rather than having one fixed action.

Estrogen is not the only reproductive hormone.

Doctors generally add a progestogen (natural progesterone or synthetic progestin) when prescribing estrogen to counteract its effect of increasing hyperplasia—an overgrowth of the uterine lining that can increase the chance of cancer. Like estrogen, a progestogen is mainly metabolized in the liver, secreted in the bile and excreted in the feces. The endogenous version can be metabolized in the brain and activates a receptor that results in varying degrees of sedation.

Because synthetic progestin is not converted in the same way, it is more likely to intensify mood disorders. Most hormone regimens commonly include synthetic progestins such as medroxyprogesterone acetate (MPA), a drug structurally related to progesterone, or norethindrone acetate, developed from the testosterone molecule. Progestins have been shown to increase breast density, and a few small studies have linked it with increasing breast cancer risk. In the uterus, however, it stops cell proliferation. There is great variation in absorption between patients. *Natural* (nature-identical or bio-identical) progesterone is sold over the counter in low doses that do not build bone or protect against hyperplasia. It is available in standardized doses by prescription from regular or compounding pharmacies. At this point the role progestins and natural progesterone play in increasing risk, when used with estrogen, continues to unfold.

The role of testosterone

Besides progestin, hormone therapies increasingly include testosterone with estrogen. Most of the testosterone a woman makes originates in the ovary and is only slightly reduced at menopause. Any drop that occurs just before or after menopause is primarily due to changes in adrenal secretion. If a woman has her ovaries removed, she may be unable to produce testosterone at suitable levels.

Two forms of exogenous testosterone are available—natural and synthetic. While most people automatically consider that "natural" makes anything better, in this case natural testosterone is poorly absorbed through the gastrointestinal tract in comparison to the synthetic version, methyltestosterone, which comes in a variety of forms including pills. Natural testosterone is available through injection or pellets, although patches are also being developed. Testosterone has specific receptors in target tissues—especially in the brain and bone. As with all the reproductive hormones, how they are utilized by an individual woman is highly variable.

LOWERED HORMONE LEVELS: THE NATURAL STATE
FOR OLDER WOMEN

So what are you to do with this information? We hope you understand that estrogen is essential to your good health. We are concerned that you use your critical thinking skills whenever it is suggested that you are hormonally *dominant* or *deficient*. When a woman's hormone levels are referred to as *estrogen dominant*, for example, it sounds as if she is so full of estrogen it should be leaking out her pores.

In truth, a woman can be estrogen dominant in her breast tissue, because of the many estrogen receptors located in the breast, while simultaneously being estrogen deficient and suffering from polycystic ovaries or severe bone loss. There are medical states and disease processes where these imbalances necessitate either the addition or exclusion of exogenous hormones. In most cases, baseline laboratory values will support such a decision.

Taking hormones at the point when your body was designed to deactivate them can stress the body, requiring it to work hard to change estrogen into breakdown products—metabolites—that are safe. In healthy women, the body persists in producing hormones at levels that are appropriate for a body that is winding down. Production continues, as we have mentioned, because the body has redundant systems. Their purpose is no longer to help you reproduce. When you go from *reproduction* to *production*, the rest of the body is fully functioning and designed to keep you going for the next thirty or forty years.

Hormone levels that are within the normal range of a menopausal woman—when you are a menopausal woman—do not dictate medicinal supplementation. Adding hormones for the purpose of restoring premenopausal levels is not what nature intended. Where is the wisdom in that? We are supposed to move beyond childbearing. Your body was designed to reproduce for three to four decades, not a lifetime. For certain the plan was not to flood it with twenty-year-old hormone levels 100 percent of the time. To that end, it is not the single-handed work of declining hormones that alone defines the progress of aging. Your *perfect design* includes getting old.

I BARELY MADE IT THROUGH THIS

There, you have it—what you need to know about hormones to become a critical thinker. If you have a headache from the details, thank God for all the new synapses you have developed! You need to know both the good and bad of estrogen and why the silver-bullet theory that hormone replacement would cure all that ails women at menopause was never a good theory—at least not for healthy women.

There should never have been a down side to any of the options a midlife woman had available to her *for the simple reason that she was not sick to begin with!* In hindsight, the risk/benefit ratio was not an appropriate way to measure the value of adding hormones. Risk to benefit analysis is fitting only when *not* intervening would result in some kind of incapacitation or accelerated mortality that could be averted by drug intervention.

Now that you think about it, are you beating yourself up for not seeing it before? Don't waste your time! Almost everyone, including advocates of "natural" and advocates of "medicalization" of menopause alike, acted under the assumption (whether they admit it or not) that menopause was a disease. Their reaction was to come up with their unique "pill for an ill." The question now is this: How are you going to apply critical thinking skills from now on?

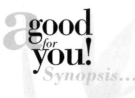

Menopause cannot be used as a scapegoat for health problems that occur as we age, and it certainly is not an excuse for ignoring them. Take a moment and ask yourself…

1. What assumptions have you made about menopause? About estrogen?

2. What symptoms have you decided are due to menopause? Are they?

3. Do you or did you believe you had to "do something" in order to get through menopause unscathed?

4. If menopause is not a disease model, what is it to you?

5. Do you see that what science knows about estrogen is an "evolving" story—one with which you must keep up?

7

what turns a good girl bad?

Fueled by the fear of estrogen, a new industry has evolved. Links on the Internet for alternatives to estrogen number in the thousands. It is the rare site that bothers to mention anything about the positive work estrogen does in the body. As the nursery rhyme laments, "when she was bad, she was horrid." Estrogen has been deemed "horrid"—and that is that. The truth, as you read in the last chapter, is that estrogen remains essential for good health throughout a woman's life span. (I might add this is so for men as well, although one doesn't often hear men "'fessing up" to their need for what is considered a "girlie" hormone!)

That such a massive effort has gone into finding substitutes or creating alternatives for estrogen is in itself a backhanded acknowledgment of its importance. But it says something else as well. The desperate search for a safe substitute (or at least another hormone that will do its work even better) continues to reinforce the assumption that without reproductive hormones a woman will be sick, shriveled or—worst yet—sick *and* shriveled!

Few authors of the thousands of Internet sites offering alternatives to estrogen grasp the reality that high levels of reproductive hormones are not needed throughout a woman's life. How we came to believe otherwise is a jumble that swirls around the wish to remain young forever, along with the belief that menopause is a disease in need of treatment.

Such assumptions are nothing new. In the early 1800s a French physician codified this belief in his book, *De la Menopause ou de l'Âge Critique des Femmes*.[1] If a woman was fortunate to live long enough to reach menopause, she would be unfortunate enough to have to face a laundry list of problems accompanied by mental deterioration. Picking up the theme, a British physician wrote in 1887 that "uterine" disease was a factor in insanity.[2] Sensing ovarian demise, he observed, ovaries at midlife send out signals that caused, if not insanity, then "extreme nervousness."[3]

My husband attended medical school during the late 1960s and remembers being taught about a psychological disorder that hits midlife women called "involutional melancholia." By 1965 the country was primed for a technological reprieve from this terrible fate. Dr. Robert Wilson's book, *Feminine Forever,* touted estrogen therapy as the proverbial fountain of youth—necessitated to counteract "the disease" of estrogen deficiency.[4]

Millions of American women and their physicians jumped on the bandwagon. To everyone's horror, ten years later the FDA warned that unopposed estrogen was associated with a 7.5 percent (and rising with longer use) increased risk of endometrial cancer. The solution, however, was already on the horizon. If estrogen was combined with a progestin, a woman's risk was actually reduced below that of someone not on hormones. Women were saved once again. Interestingly, it is this combination twenty-seven years later that is the subject of the current controversy over hormone replacement therapy.

something *to* *think about*

There was a little girl
  who had a little curl
Right in the middle of her
  forehead;
When she was good,
  she was very, very good,
And when she was bad,
  she was horrid.[5]

In the 1990s, a number of books were written that unbolted the door to an open discussion of menopause. While the perception of menopause as disease was beginning to be challenged, most conversations focused on the misery and disruption of the transition. Writings about women becoming independent, rearranging their lives and being happy were chiefly found among more fringe audiences. Neither being sick nor being wizened is particularly appealing.

PASSING THE TESTS

While hormones came to the attention of physicians in the 1930s, it wasn't until the 1960s that replenishing them at midlife became the treatment of choice. The most widely used estrogen, Premarin, was approved in 1942. Its acceptance by the Food and Drug Administration (FDA) was based on satisfactory chemistry and manufacturing plus reports from clinical trials that the drug was safe for its intended use, which was defined as treatment of menopausal symptoms and related conditions.

onsider *this...* The National Institutes of Health have added steroidal estrogens and oral contraceptives to their list of known human carcinogens (cancer-causing agents).[6]

The introduction of Premarin predated the current requirements for comprehensive analysis of every component in any product under review. No one at the time knew everything it contained, and therefore, testing what each component did was not possible. The thinking of the day was that most estrogens could be judged by their final potency and that everything in them worked to that end. Today researchers know that not all estrogens or progestogens work the same way, and therefore may not be interchangeable. Even the method of delivery (in what form you take them) makes them different.

It is interesting to note that in 1997 a generic form of Premarin was turned down by the FDA because all the ingredients and their exact mechanism of action had still not been defined and therefore could not be duplicated. In 1990, Wyeth, the company that produces Premarin, petitioned the FDA for new labeling that went beyond relief of menopausal symptoms to include cardiovascular protection. The FDA asked for proof, so Wyeth initiated a well-designed double-blind, randomized, placebo-controlled clinical trial, the Heart and Estrogen/Progestin Replacement Study (HERS).[7]

To everyone's dismay and totally opposite of the conventional wisdom of the medical profession, no significant overall difference in the occurrence of cardiovascular disease was noted, despite 10–11 percent drops in low-density lipoprotein (LDL–the bad cholesterol) and equivalent increases in HDL (the good cholesterol). The follow-up HERS II study was designed to determine if HRT provided cardiovascular protection for older women who already suffered from heart disease. The unexpected conclusion was that such women were at *increased* risk, especially if they were just starting an HRT regime.

The black eye that HRT received from the two HERS studies was nothing compared to the knockout punch of the Women's Health Initiative. Simply stated, analysis of all the information revealed that for every ten thousand women receiving estrogen/progestin (HRT) therapy (Prempro or Premphase), there will be eight more breast cancers, eight more strokes, seven more heart attacks, eighteen more venous-thrombotic events, six fewer colon cancers and five fewer hip fractures than among women not receiving HRT.[8]

More recent analysis of data from the HERS study found that women on estrogen and progestin with no urinary incontinence at baseline (average age sixty-six, eighteen years past menopause) found a twofold increase in urge incontinence and fourfold increase in stress incontinence. The risk of developing the disorders increased with time.[9]

Sizzle over science

How did it happen that a drug regimen was so universally accepted when no previous controlled trials had ever shown definitively that HRT prevented cardiovascular disease, stroke, Alzheimer's or even wrinkles? This is an interesting question when contemplated in context of the medical community's almost universal cry against the use of botanicals and supplements for lack of proof as measured by double-blind, placebo-controlled studies. Ignoring two thousand years of effective and safe use of many natural products is an interesting omission.

Doctors became believers in HRT without proof of its efficacy. How did that happen? As women, we cannot absolve our role. The promise and hope of "feminine forever," "youthful evermore," a "pill for an ill" are strong motivations to beat a hasty path to the nearest doctor's office. We see the same behavior with Allegra (allergies), Prilosec (acid reflux) and Meridian (weight loss). Prompted by the mix of science and advertising on television, the "direct-to-consumer" appeal, served in equal doses with our morning coffee, results in demands for prescriptions.

That said, clearly the greatest influence came about because the drug companies told physicians that HRT was a good thing. You may be unaware that drug companies are responsible for most of the post-medical-school-education a physician receives. With the overwhelming task of keeping up on the latest technology, it is natural for doctors to seek the bottom line, the summary version. But this is a dangerous practice.

Researchers funded by the drug company, for instance, gave presentations at conferences that reinterpreted the HERS study to say there was benefit from HRT, it just took a while, ignoring that cumulative cardiovascular events were similar between the treated and control groups. The new logic went so far as to state that because women had earlier cardiovascular events, they were saved from having them later, and that if they got breast cancer, it was less deadly if they had taken HRT. They insisted that those in HERS II who already had cardiovascular disease were simply too sick to get the benefit; women who were healthy would be helped by HRT. Obviously, no one listening to such explanations was doing much critical thinking!

The numerous studies demonstrating that women who took estrogen had fewer cardiovascular events is likely explained by what some researchers suspected all along: HRT users have been shown to have fewer health risks in the first place and are more likely to take care of themselves. Apparently HRT is more of a marker for less heart disease, not a player in its reduction.[10]

onsider *this...* According to the Women's Health Initiative, risk of pulmonary embolism (blood clots in lungs) rises shortly after starting HRT; stroke risk increases after the first year; invasive breast cancer rates begin to rise the fourth year.[11]

The withdrawal of HRT as the main "fix" for "women of a certain age" has created a plethora of "What Now?" articles in medical and lay journals. I'm sorry to say that some articles in professional journals don't sound much more hopeful than those from the 1800s. The president of the American Association of Obstetricians and Gynecologists wrote in the September 15, 2002 issue of *OBGyn News*, "It is too soon for us to give opinions and advice while we are facing this tidal wave of negativism from both the press and the public...My advice to patients is there's no urgency to make a change. Let's have a debate nationally and then decide what we as physicians are going to recommend and implement..."

I hope you recognize by now that trying to avoid upset and decision making by consensus are not techniques of critical thinking. And where does a patient's viewpoint fit in such a plan?

The observation has been made that the fallout from the WHI study will be a *defining* moment for gynecologists. The scramble is on for a replacement. One article speaks of trials already underway to consider HRT and SERM use together as "the perfect ticket, but time will tell."[12] Others pin hopes on lower doses, new methods of delivery and different formulations—even a return to straight estrogen is being suggested. The lack of serious discussion of botanicals and of improving overall health as a means of reducing menopause symptomology is striking.

> **T**hink about *it* ... Therapies given to a healthy population must be held to a higher standard of safety than therapies used to treat disease ... Persuading the medical community that healthy asymptomatic women should take hormones as a health-promoting tonic was a brilliant and profitable move on the part of pharmaceutical companies.[13]

HOW ESTROGEN GOES BAD

Depending on external and internal influences, estrogen will behave well or potentially cause serious damage. While your genes will play a part in how estrogen interacts with your cells, their expression is skewed by many factors. The chance they will give an order for cancer or some other disease process depends to a large extent on multiple dynamics, many of which are under your control.

For our brief discussion, you need to understand that the "good girl" estrogen is represented by the symbol 2-OH; bad estrogen is expressed as 4-OH and 16-OH.

Keeping a good girl *good*

Since estrogen is broken down in the liver, it makes sense that healthy liver function is important. The liver's role includes "detoxification," which means it takes something that can harm us and changes it into a form that is no longer dangerous. If your liver is working as it should, it can minimize, through detoxification and excretion, production of highly reactive breakdown products of estrogen that can damage DNA and trigger cancer directly or indirectly. Trouble also results when pathogenic gut bacteria in an unbalanced intestine allow estrogen to reenter the circulation. Bad guy bacteria are associated with greater cancer risk, including breast cancer. This threat is increased by a diet high in fat and low in fiber.

D id you know? An agonist is estrogen-like, while an antagonist opposes estrogen action.

The role of phytoestrogens and other natural nutrients

Phytoestrogens found in a wide variety of plant foods (legumes, clover, soy, kudzu, alfalfa, licorice root) can act like an estrogen or an antiestrogen, depending on what the body needs. In essence, the isoflavones and lignans they contain are nature's SERMs.[14] Their roles are as adaptogens—estrogen agonist and antagonist—and they involve themselves in different signaling and gene processes. Research confirms that increased isoflavone consumption leads to favorable metabolite ratios and decreased estrogen production. The following are favorable effects some of these nutrients provide:

- Resveratrol is found in many plants but is especially plentiful in grapes. It has its own special estrogen-modulating effects that lower breast cell proliferation and influence circulating estrogen.[15] New studies suggest grape juice has plenty of healthful properties should you not care to imbibe your medicine as red wine.[16] Lignans (found in flaxseeds, the bran layer of grains, beans and seeds) and isoflavones (like soy and red clover) are converted in the colon to a biologically active form that in turn affects the production of hormones. Prompting a shift to 2-OH metabolites (good-girl estrogen) is one of the most important things soy does. The presence of appropriate bacteria in a favorable balance is an essential part of the metabolic work.

  A person who has eaten soy for a lifetime is apt to have the proper ratio of bacteria and might gain significantly more than someone who has added soy to their diet only recently. In other words, it is not only what you eat, but also the mechanism to convert the food into a usable, effective form that is important.

- Genetic variations can make you more susceptible to producing 4-OH or 16-OH metabolites (bad-girl estrogen). Low levels of B vitamins (B$_6$, B$_{12}$ and folate) interrupt proper estrogen detoxification, resulting in increased estrogen. A significant percentage of the population have problems utilizing B-vitamin folate (folic acid), placing them at risk for higher levels of homocysteine and consequent peril for stroke and cardiovascular disease, depression, Alzheimer's and colon and breast cancer. The problem is solved with biologically active forms of folate (5-formyl tetrahydrofolate and 5-methyl tetrahydrofolate).

- Antioxidants such as green tea and D-limonene (from citrus fruits) prevent the formation of very reactive breakdown products of estrogen, important because they directly and negatively affect DNA.

- It is known that dietary intake of indole-3-carbinol (broccoli, cabbage and other cruciferous vegetables) is protective because of its ability to influence positively liver function to excrete estrogen and to promote "good-girl" estrogen metabolites. If you prefer your vegetables in pill form, two different extracts from cruciferous vegetables known as indole-3-carbinol and diindolylmethane (DIM) are roughly equivalent to eating two pounds of broccoli.

- Watch the fats! The balance, amount and type of fats consumed can be critical as well. Breast cancer cells exposed to omega-3 fatty acid from cold-water fish have a favorable 2-OH ratio (good girl) in laboratory research.[17] Inadequate levels of protein may lead to liver detoxification problems, as do low levels of vitamin E.

- In the laboratory, vitamin E has been shown to inhibit growth of breast cancer cells.

- Magnesium is important for breakdown and excretion of estrogen.

- Finally, research confirms that naturally occurring spices such as curcumin from the curry spice and turmeric, a member of the ginger family, can be particularly effective in protecting against environmentally toxic estrogens that stimulate growth on receptor positive and negative breast cancer cells. They also enhance detoxification.

Obesity weighs in

Inherited genetic propensity and obesity each have their own ways of escalating cancer risk. Obesity is a problem because it provides extra fat cells for estrogen production. Getting down to your ideal weight means that you have reduced the territory where estrogen can be made. Additionally, too much insulin in the bloodstream prompts the ovaries to secrete excess testosterone and in turn reduces sex-hormone-binding globulin (SHBG) levels, freeing estrogen to do its damage. The decision to lose weight, if you have added some baby fat to your grown-up frame, is an excellent first choice in any effort made to reduce the chance of having your estrogen misbehave.

Think about *it* ... Women with more 2-OH have been shown to be 40 percent less likely to get breast cancer. A 30 percent reduction in cancer risk is found in women with the highest 2-OH ratios versus those with the lowest.[18]

Consumption of alcohol

For those who decide to drink alcoholic beverages instead of eat, the news is not good. Estrogen levels are increased with alcohol consumption of more than 12 ounces of beer, 5 ounces of wine or 1.5 ounces of 80-proof distilled spirits per day. Breast cancer risk is notably escalated when alcohol is combined with HRT.[19]

Estrogen imposters

If you have been paying attention, you have noticed that, after taking into account your genes, lowering disease risk linked to bad-girl estrogen is significantly dependent on what you eat, how fit and trim you are, and, we must add, environmental exposure to toxins and exogenous hormones of various types. Numerous pesticides, carcinogens, certain drugs like cyclosporine and cimetedine (Tagamet), can cause the metabolite ratio to tilt in favor of developing cancer. This is because so many environmental toxins have structures so similar to estrogen, they can mimic detrimental estrogen metabolites. No matter the source, many are capable of binding to estrogen receptors.

Environmental estrogens are known as ecoestrogens or xenoestrogens. Innumerable natural and synthetic organic compounds can duplicate estrogen's actions—with the exception of stimulating a reproductive cycle. The result can be a normal response, an abnormal one or simply interference with normal hormone binding. Unlike phytoestrogens from food that break down and spend little time in the body, synthetic environmental estrogens linger on the receptors, increasing the potential for harm.

Examples include aromatic hydrocarbons and organochlorines found in pesticides, herbicides, plastics, refrigerants, industrial solvents and many household products. The chemical p-nonylphenol (NP), used to harden the PVC plastic of water and sewage pipes and used to strengthen containers that hold water, milk and juice, has been found to be estrogenic.[20] There are legitimate concerns about the hormones used to fatten livestock and promote milk production. We know a considerable amount about how these chemicals can alter an animal's life cycle and health. We don't know the full extent of their effect on humans. We must assume that length of exposure, the dose, age, health and individual genetic diversity make a difference in how much harm is done.

TO BE CONTINUED . . .

The unfolding estrogen story is about the form and the messages conveyed by estrogen as it continually passes through the body. To a great extent, it is food that makes the difference between harmful and favorable messages. Food is the buffer that can enhance your health or work against you. It becomes powerful medicine when combined with your genes. You have reason to question the value of processed foods, additives and your food sources.

Does this begin to make you think that every meal counts? Do you want to be in control of the DNA conversation? Parents that don't require boundaries for their children increase the odds of poor behavior and practically insure it if there is a genetic propensity to violence. When it comes to our personal health, we are sometimes "poor parents." Our good-girl/bad-girl hormone "children" run free when we do not monitor and set limits. We are good parents when what we eat becomes important.

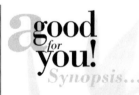
a **good** *for* **you!** *Synopsis...*

Whew! This is a big concept.
1. Did you process it correctly?
2. Do you understand what a metabolite is?
3. Is it clear the numerous ways you can influence the work of your hormones?
4. What can you do to be a better "parent" of your hormones?
5. Do you understand that simply by shifting your food choices even slightly in favor of more vegetables like broccoli and brussel sprouts and less "empty-calorie" treats every day enlivens your body and protects you from cancer?

PART II
The Baseline

Before you begin to make meaningful changes to maximize your well-being now and to ensure healthy aging in the future, you must be clear about your current health—not what you would like it to be or think it is, but an unblinking assessment of how you are doing.

To help you, chapter eight contains suggestions and laboratory tests for gathering information that will enable you to design a path that maximizes your optimal health and vitality.

Since you are likely to require a doctor's advice and help, chapter nine will give you tools to help enlist your health practitioner as your health partner.

Chapters ten and eleven present the foundational table on which to begin: sound nutrition, exercise and coping effectively with stress. These are your baseline elements—ignoring them will take years off your life and lessen your pleasure in it.

8

knowing your baseline

There are some aspects of staying healthy that don't sound like much fun. If we followed every suggestion that drifts into our living rooms over the television news or in our magazines, our time would be spent organizing what we believe we must learn to do *with* or *without*. Take heart if you feel overwhelmed. Most of what you need to do to attain your optimal health requires *simplification,* not complication. Efforts at maintaining wellness are not supposed to make you sick!

How do you make staying healthy fun or, minimally at least, not a pity party? The good news is that if you live life in a way that you are able to do—what you must do and what you want to do—good practices reinforce themselves. Things like choosing simply prepared fresh, colorful food, adopting a lifestyle that leaves time for fun, for doing nothing and for cultivation of loving relationships with people who also know how to love are all good practices.

Living healthy is not about becoming afraid that eating something that is not organic or contains "bad" fat necessitates picking out songs for your funeral. It does not require never taking another drink out of a plastic bottle (especially one you have frozen) or no longer going out for fear of inhaling someone's secondhand smoke. It is about aging gracefully and with vitality. It is about common sense.

It is wonderful to know that many options that lead to health are under your direct control. That means that you alone can have a powerful impact on continuing to work at a job you love, playing a sport you adore or beginning each day raring to meet whatever comes along. Living what has been referred to as a "therapeutic" lifestyle is not that difficult. You already know the basics—learning how to tweak a few things for your particular issues may be all that is necessary.

But know this, living "therapeutically" will influence everything from your energy level and hormone balance to your vulnerability to serious and chronic diseases like diabetes and heart disease. That said, a therapeutic lifestyle does require reality checks. First, you must gather information to be certain about the current state of your health, not what you think it is, but as close as possible to your true condition. You must not start with biased assumptions.

something
to think about

What you prevent you don't have to cure.

The information you gather can be used to discriminate between menopause symptomology and serious illness, between what we frequently accept as aging and actual illness—especially the degenerative and chronic illnesses that begin long before they make their presence known. As we mentioned, they may have had their nidus in your thirties—way back when you were looking good—and can begin making life uncomfortable around menopause. If degenerative diseases are ignored and dismissed as "menopause" complaints, their progressive decline continues, gains momentum and ends up as a disability so severe that you require your children to parent you. If that thought makes you shudder, then perhaps you will be open to instituting some changes that can prevent or push back such a scenario. *Good for you*—and keep reading.

WHERE DO YOU START?

Even with the best of intentions, well-formulated products and your knowledge, you are likely to fail to ensure wellness if you are *guessing* about the state of your overall health. If you are serious about good health and want to live a therapeutic lifestyle, then you must "bite the bullet" and have some tests done. A hit-or-miss approach to healing and wellness can leave real undiagnosed medical issues untreated, cause increased harm, be very expensive and, in the end, do nothing to improve your overall fitness despite a great deal of effort, attention and money. Your first step to action is *knowing your* baseline.

Even if you are not fond of your conventional practitioner, chances are you will need him or her to order laboratory tests, help interpret them and make recommendations based on their results. Laboratory tests should always be ordered and interpreted in consideration of the following:

- Your personal health history
- Your family history
- Your lifestyle practices
- Your philosophy about the use of natural and conventional interventions
- Your finances and insurance
- Your "personal" index of suspicions (how you actually feel and subtle changes you notice)

onsider *this...*   Risk factors for diseases of aging are high blood pressure, abnormal cholesterol metabolism, high or low thyroid levels, high insulin levels, increased body fat (particularly around the waist) and/or increasing loss of strength.

Enlisting a medical practitioner to order tests for you does not absolve you of responsibility. You must be aware of the tests your practitioner should be ordering. You need to have a general idea as to why and when they may be necessary—especially in light of your personal history. In this day of cost cutting, it is unlikely that your practitioner will add tests that are not necessary. It is more likely that after reading *Good for You!* you may request some tests with which he or she is unfamiliar.

But remember, test results outside of a context are of minimal value. Do your homework and find out as much as possible about your family and your health history as a child. What serious illnesses have relatives suffered; what did they die from and at what age? Age is significant with breast cancer and heart attacks because genetic risk will vary depending on when they occurred. Your own health history and lifestyle are relevant in analyzing and deciding what to do with test results.

SOME TESTS TO CONSIDER (OR NOT)

If you study the following charts carefully, you will become informed regarding what tests are available and which you should consider in order to determine your current state of health.

Hormone tests can measure individual hormones of many types, including FSH, testosterone, estrogen and progesterone. A good test includes FSH, estrogen and progesterone at least. The result can be measures of each one individually, which has certain clinical relevance. If FSH measures in a certain level, we can draw conclusions about menopause.

measurements of hormones

WHY?	HOW?	WHO?	RESULTS?
Measures estradiol, estrone, estriol, proges- terone and testos- terone levels and their ratios of one to the other; follic- ular stimulating hormone (FSH) and sex-hormone- binding globulin (SHBG) levels	Saliva or blood; urine not as accu- rate; five- or twenty-eight-day saliva avoids "snapshot" effect; time of menstrual cycle relevant	Pre- and peri- menopausal women to rule out early menopause as a contributing factor to depres- sion, weight gain, etc.; pre- menopause, to improve ovarian function if experi- encing infertility, painful or erratic periods; premature menopause	Not much rele- vance in peri- menopause; possible baseline for comparison; FSH above 40 sig- nals menopause; FSH = 20 signals symptoms. Perimenopause results: preovula- tory = 1.5–11.4 MIU/ml (milli inter- national units per milliliter); ovulatory = 5.1–34.2 MIU/ml; postovula- tory = 27.6–132.9 MIU/ml

Comment: Almost every woman who came to A Woman's Place, my husband's clinic, for issues of menopause expected and/or requested that her "hormone" levels be tested. It proved difficult to convince her she might not benefit from the information derived. Because the nature of peri- menopause is one of great hormonal flux, capturing test results that mean something can be difficult.

Most women merely confirm what is an obvious certainty of menopause—that hormones are produced at lower levels and they are "estrogen dominant." This is because menstrual cycles at menopause often occur without ovulation. When an egg is not released, progesterone pro- duction is reduced. This is normal for menopausal women. The truth is there are no standardized baseline levels of reproductive hormones that are correct for all women. Nevertheless, many women use such levels in com- bination with other factors to help confirm their menopausal state.

estrogen metabolism assessment

WHY?	HOW?	WHO?	RESULTS?
Measures the ratio and levels of 2-OH and 16-OH estrogen metabolites.	Either blood or urine; premenopause: days 19–25 of period; women on HRT or oral contraceptives: 8–10 hours after their last dose.	Any with estrogen-dependent health problems such as breast cancer, lupus, osteoporosis and heart disease; women who want a baseline from which to monitor the effectiveness of dietary, lifestyle and hormone therapies.	The imbalance of estrogen metabolites can lead to serious health problems, including cancer.

Comment: While this is an FDA-approved test, it is unlikely it will be on your local laboratory's panel. In our opinion, this test is at least as valuable as measuring hormone levels, perhaps more so. Because metabolite production can be influenced by paying attention to diet and lifestyle, results provide a baseline that can give a woman motivation to begin or maintain positive intervention.

Measurements for cardiovascular disease risk

The following tests when considered together give a picture of your cardiovascular risk.

high sensitivity c-reactive protein (CRP)

WHY?	HOW?	WHO?	RESULTS?
Relatively inexpensive test to detect increases in inflammation processes.	Blood sample—insist on high sensitivity CRP.	All menopausal women as a baseline.	Elevated CRP is predictive of cardiovascular risk apart from LDL measurements and increases risk of a heart attack 4.5 times; normal levels should be under 0.11 mg per deciliter of blood (mg/dL).

Comment: While there is controversy as to the appropriateness of using the CRP test as a general screening device, midlife is a perfect time for such a test. High levels require follow-up because they indicate inflammation processes for various diseases. Besides being a marker for heart attack, it is also relevant for stroke, high blood pressure and arterial disease. A woman with "intermediate risk" for heart disease, meaning a 10–20 percent chance within ten years, because of elevated CRP levels may opt to be treated more aggressively. CRP is a better predictor of a heart attack than levels of cholesterol or homocysteine. Women with metabolic syndrome, linked to obesity and a potential for diabetes, will have high CRP levels. CRP levels are very sensitive to diet, exercise and losing weight; therefore, the test can provide motivation for making therapeutic lifestyle changes.

homocysteine

WHY?	HOW?	WHO?	RESULTS?
High levels cause damage to the walls of blood vessels, increasing the chance of cholesterol deposits.	Blood sample.	Those with a diet high in red meat; vegetarians; any with problems with B_{12} metabolism, family history of heart disease or kidney problems.	Ideal: 5–7 micromoles per liter of blood (mmol/L); above 13 mmol/L indicates a high probability of an active disease process.

Comment: Homocysteine is a normal by-product of protein metabolism. Some people carry genes that interfere with the ability of folic acid to lower homocysteine levels. (See the information on Cardio Genomic Profile in Appendix A.) If your diet is high in red meat and your intake of vitamins B_6 and B_{12} is low, you are apt to have elevated homocysteine. Vegetarians can also have high homocysteine if they have low B_{12} levels.

lipid profile

WHY?	HOW?	WHO?	RESULTS?
Levels of the various cholesterols are related to cardiovascular risk.	Blood sample; insist on a complete panel: overall cholesterol, triglycerides, low-density lipoprotein (LDL) and high-density lipoprotein (HDL); if possible, very-low-density lipoproteins (VLDL) and lipoproteins A and B.	A baseline for everyone; more frequent monitoring with family history or elevated rates.	Refer to Table #1.

table 1

CHOLESTEROL	DESIRABLE
LDL (mg/dL)	Below 130
HDL (mg/dL)	Above 40
VLDL (mg/dL) Total Cholesterol/ HDL Ratio LDL/HDL Ratio	Below 20 Less than 5.0 Less than 3.2
Total Cholesterol (mg/dL)	Less than 200

Comment: The ratios of one cholesterol to another give a more accurate risk assessment than any one number. The worst case would be high total cholesterol, triglycerides and LDL. HDL should be one-third or more of the total cholesterol. High triglycerides and low HDL are problematic. VLDL and lipoproteins A and B are relatively new but recommended because they reveal risks not always evident with the "usual" lipids. If your cholesterol is within the normal range, but members of your family have heart disease, make sure you include them because these measures tend to pick up heritability.

blood pressure

WHY?	HOW?	WHO?	RESULTS?
Measure of the ability of blood vessels to stretch and adjust to normal fluctuations in blood flow; high pressure increases heart disease and stroke.	Blood pressure cuff around the arm or finger device.	Anyone with extra weight, kidney or heart problems, diabetes or of black ethnicity.	Risk begins to increase at 115/75.

Comment: As pressure and stress increase, damage is done to blood vessel walls leaving them susceptible to cholesterol buildup as well as kidney damage. Easy-to-read blood pressure measuring devices are readily available at most pharmacies or drug stores. An estimated fifty million people have high blood pressure (hypertension). High blood pressure coupled with elevated insulin levels (common with diabetes and obesity) must be carefully controlled to avoid increasing heart disease. Persistent high blood pressure is significant; a few sporadic high blood pressure measurements are not.

Glucose testing

It is also important to include a test to measure glucose when considering your cardiovascular disease risk. Please refer to the chart on page 81 for measurement of blood sugar levels.

It has long been known that diabetics who experience increased levels of blood sugar (glucose) are at risk for heart disease. It is now believed that even small but chronic increases put a person at risk. Excess insulin, the response to high sugar levels in the blood, raises cholesterol and blood pressure.

Measurement of thyroid function

Thyroid imbalance is a "menopause imposter" because its symptoms mimic those of the "change." Making the distinction is critical. Women with complaints of general "un-wellness," fatigue, depression, coldness, constipation, dry skin, headaches, PMS, fluid retention, weight gain, anxiety/panic attacks, memory and/or concentration problems, muscle/joint pain and low sex drive may find their complaints related to an unbalanced thyroid.

thyroid

WHY?	HOW?	WHO?	RESULTS?
Increase in thyroid imbalance at midlife; mimics menopause symptoms; far-reaching health damage if ignored.	Blood sample; thyroid-stimulating hormone (TSH); unbound levels of thyroxine (T4), tri-iodothyronine (T3); other tests: bioactive portion of thyroid, auto-immune reactions and altered peripheral conversion of T3.	Baseline for all women and those with complaints of fatigue, coldness, weight gain, memory problems.	A TSH should fall in a normal range of .75–5.5.

Comment: If your doctor insists you test in the low but "normal" range, consider a month trial of an appropriate medication anyway. Thyroid testing is likely to measure a "point in time" versus what is usual for you. Ignoring thyroid imbalance can profoundly affect your metabolic balance, utilization of carbohydrates, fats, vitamins, cell energy, hormone secretion and more. If the usual thyroid dose restores you to a "normal" range but not to feeling well, more comprehensive testing is called for.

Tests for osteoporosis

It is not difficult to determine your risk for osteoporosis. The DXA test releases minimal radiation, takes less than twenty minutes and doesn't require that you remove your clothes!

osteoporosis

WHY?	HOW?	WHO?	RESULTS?
The exact condition of your bones can be calculated. Osteoporosis risk increases the first five years after periods stop. This is a preventable disease in most cases.	The gold standard is a DXA (Dual X-ray Absorptiometry). Wrist and heel bone screening can be used to see if a DXA is necessary.	Menopausal women; family history; history of an eating disorder; low calcium ingestion as teen; steroid use (for arthritis or asthma); lack of or extreme exercise (marathon runner, ballet dancer); all women by age sixty-five; earlier for white or Asian women with one risk factor; any midlife or older woman who breaks a bone.	The DXA compares your results with other women your age and against younger women.

Comment: Do not bother with more potent and less accurate x-ray measures. Quantitative Computed Tomography (QCT) and Quantitative Ultrasound (QUS) are reliable for measuring baseline bone mass and estimating fracture risk, but lack the precision of DXA for tracking the success of therapy.

You may have noticed that your pharmacy or a health fair offers bone-density tests (QUS) that take wrist or foot readings. These are very reasonably priced (often around 25 dollars) and are good for preliminary screening to determine if a DXA is needed. Special urine and blood tests can be used in between DXA testing to determine if treatment interventions are working.

Measurements of blood sugar levels

Tests of blood sugar (glucose) determine how well your body metabolizes your sugar and other carbohydrates. Early assessments of imbalances are important because therapeutic lifestyle interventions are effective.

glucose

WHY?	HOW?	WHO?	RESULTS?
Even small but chronic increases in blood sugar put a person at risk for heart disease, diabetes and weight control problems that undermine well-being.	Blood sample is taken after a twelve-hour fast or more accurate two-hour post-challenge glucose and insulin level test; a glycated hemoglobin (HbA1c) blood test measures blood sugar over a two-week span.	Any who are overweight, particularly with fat accumulation around the middle.	Fasting two-hour post-challenge glucose and insulin level test: 70–111 mg/dL are normal, 75–85 mg/dL is healthier; a 50 mg/dL change in one hour indicates a prediabetic state. Normal range hemoglobin A1c is 4.7–6.4.

Comment: Metabolic changes that can lead to diabetes can be picked up ten or more years before the disease shows itself. Obviously, anyone diagnosed with diabetes must monitor her blood sugar carefully. It is estimated that one out of every three adults has some problems handling the sugar in his system, overweight or not. Besides giving a baseline for response to treatment, a healthy glucose (sugar) balance results in an improved cardiovascular condition, more energy, better moods, easier weight maintenance and healthier aging.

Colorectal cancer testing

In the next few years testing for colon cancer via a simple blood test will be available. For now, a colonoscopy is an outpatient procedure performed on a cleansed bowel under an intravenous (IV) twilight anesthesia and pain medication. A scope attached to a flexible tube capable of reaching the entire colon is introduced, and images of your colon are projected on a screen.

colon cancer testing

WHY?	HOW?	WHO?	RESULTS?
Colon cancer increases as we age but is treatable if caught early.	Fecal occult blood tests and colonoscopy.	Baseline at midlife and those with a family history.	Blood in the stool requires further testing; visual examination reveals the health of the colon.

Comment: A baseline colonoscopy is recommended at age fifty and should be repeated every five to ten years depending on history. If polyps (potentially cancerous growths) are found during the colonoscopy, most can be removed at the time, eliminating the need for a second procedure. Laboratory evaluation reveals whether polyps are benign or malignant.

Adrenocortex measurements

A circadian analysis of cortisol activity gives vital information about sleep and energy peaks and valleys. Overproduction of cortisol wears the body down and leads to premature aging, heart disease and lowered immunity.

adrenocortex stress profile

WHY?	HOW?	WHO?	RESULTS?
Measurements evaluate the bioavailability and level of cortisol, and DHEA baselines indicate the effectiveness of interventions.	Saliva samples over twenty-four hours.	Women with complaints of fatigue, sleep problems and anxiety.	Reported graphically; interpretation is by the testing laboratory. (See Appendix A.)

Comments: DHEA is a good indicator of adrenal function. It is produced from pregnenolone and converted into testosterone, estrone and estradiol. Many women suffer "adrenal burnout" at menopause. Improving adrenal function frequently improves menopausal symptomology. (See Appendix A.)

AND WHAT ABOUT...

General measurements of blood chemistry

Blood chemistry panels measure levels of a multitude of factors including calcium, sodium, potassium, enzymes, bilirubin and electrolytes, just to name a few. The panel can include glucose and lipid screens that are sensitive enough to indicate levels that require more sophisticated testing.

Pap tests

It is a good idea to get an annual Pap test, although increasingly it is being recommended every two or three years if you have had three normal Pap tests in a row. Pap tests were developed to detect cervical cancer, but they can also pick up infections, inflammation and abnormal cells that may become cancer. Whether women who have had hysterectomies need a Pap test depends on the type of surgery—although a pelvic exam is still in order.

Do not douche, use suppositories, foams or vaginal medications at least two days before the test. Refrain from sexual intercourse for twenty-four hours. If you still have menstrual periods, schedule an appointment between the tenth and twentieth days of your cycle and never during a period.

A stick, swab or brush is used to dislodge a few cells from the cervical area, placed on a slide and interpreted at a laboratory. Since the test is not 100 percent accurate, it is repeated if results are other than normal. Ongoing research on FDA-approved but newer (and more expensive) tests such as the Thin-Prep Pap Test, PAPNET and the AutoPap300QC will determine if they are more accurate than the original version.

Mammogram

The problem with mammograms is not whether or not they are effective at detecting early evidence of breast cancer—they *are*. The controversy is over when a woman should start having them. There is no disagreement with beginning to have mammograms at age fifty.

Those who do not recommend their use in forty- to forty-nine-year-olds maintain that "abnormal" growths subject women to invasive procedures for prevention they may have never needed. Scientists who recommend earlier mammograms maintain that women have smaller tumors, less chance of spread and more breast conservation than those who wait. Insurance companies are increasingly paying for double reads, either by a second technician or a computer.

Computerized Thermal Imaging (CTI) picks up increased heat radiated by cancer cells and is showing promise in differentiating between normal and suspicious spots, thus reducing the number of biopsies. Research continues while it awaits FDA approval.

Ductal lavage is FDA approved and is much like a Pap test, seeking to collect cells "that are thinking about becoming cancer." Cells are extracted from the milk ducts. Ductal lavage is intended to be used in conjunction with mammograms. "Precancerous" cells give a woman a heads-up choice about preventative treatment. Being familiar with your own breasts and your usual set of lumps and bumps versus any new ones is equally important. That said, keep in mind that needle biopsies make diagnosis much less invasive than before by aspirating a few cells into a syringe.

Note: The U.S. Preventive Services Task Force advises women in their forties to start mammograms.

Think about *it*... In a fifteen year study involving 250,000 fifty-five- to seventy-year-old women, mammography reduced breast cancer deaths by 21 percent compared to the control group.[1]

The September 3, 2002 issue of the *Annals of Internal Medicine* reported that the Canadian National Breast Screening Study of over 50,000 forty- to forty-nine-year-old women revealed those who got mammograms were just as likely to die from breast cancer as those who did not, even though earlier and more cancers were detected. The study results became statistically relevant after eleven to sixteen years.

Tests for Alzheimer's Disease

In the past, Alzheimer's disease was said to be undiagnosable until autopsy. Today "brain-imaging" techniques are so sophisticated they actually watch the brain at work.

Magnetic Resonance Imaging (MRI) technology enables a 3-D view of the minute structures of the brain, including those that are damaged. Positron-Emission Tomography (PET) scans captured images of the brain in motion, measuring working memory. Functional Magnetic Resonance (FMR) monitors changes in the brain by how much oxygen is being consumed while a patient is remembering and repeating words presented to them. Magneto-Encephalography (MEG) shows the brain at work by measuring nerve-cell firing, indicating the order and sequence of the working brain.

What all this means is that there are very sophisticated techniques available that reveal patterns characteristic of dementia. Perhaps more importantly, they are capable of discerning minute changes of mild cognitive impairment, a pre-Alzheimer's condition that, if recognized early, is amenable to a number of medications that prolong the onset of Alzheimer's disease.

Genetic testing

Until recently, testing for genes that increased one's chance for Alzheimer's or breast cancer was somewhat of a no-win proposition. If you found you were a carrier, there was nothing you could do. Today, early intervention and a number of options are possible for high-risk situations.

Sometimes just knowing one has a propensity for disease becomes motivation to follow good health practices. Ultimately, the decision becomes an informed one made between a woman and her doctor.

AND DON'T FORGET...

An annual eye exam

Three eye diseases increase as we age: macular degeneration, glaucoma and cataracts. You may be experiencing macular degeneration if your vision seems dim or distorted, especially when you try to focus, or if you experience blank spots. A professional can determine if you have this disease by an eye examination.

Glaucoma occurs as the result of undetectable increasing pressure in the eye, which is detected by an opthamological machine. Early diagnosis diminishes its progression by half.

Cataracts, which can result in severe visual impairment, can also be diagnosed during an opthamalogic exam.

A dental exam

A thorough exam by a dentist involves more than cleaning your teeth and giving you a new toothbrush. A good dentist will also evaluate skin conditions on the face, lumps in the neck area and on the inside of the mouth.

Caution: If you have been diagnosed with mitral-valve prolapse, you must take an antibiotic one hour prior to having your teeth cleaned or repaired. Do not take this caution lightly!

Dermatological exam

Like other illnesses that wait until you are older to rear their unattractive head, skin problems escalate at midlife. While it is important to keep an eye on any skin changes yourself, a good dermatologist is likely to see problems you might overlook. Those with fair skin or who mistakenly assume a tan is as healthy as it looks may need to be on a more frequent schedule. Wear a hat and use sunscreen.

Were you *wondering*? Waist circumference over thirty-five inches increases risk for cardiovascular disease. Ultrasound measurements of intra-abdominal fat are even more accurate in diagnosing metabolic syndrome.[2]

THE MIRROR TEST

There is no question that each of these tests will reveal valuable information about your baseline health. Depending on your insurance policy, many of the tests will be covered. Should you find that finances are limiting your opportunity to have some of these tests, there are things you can do on your own. The first is the "mirror, mirror on the wall" test. It costs nothing except a bit of nerve.

An honest evaluation of your weight and how you are carrying it is apparent by taking a good look. If your figure looks more like an apple than a classic hourglass, you need to know that you are at greater risk for heart disease and diabetes. You can use the Internet to calculate your body mass index (BMI), a number that categorizes your weight as overweight (25–29.9), obese (above 30) or underweight (18.5 or less). Check www.webMD.com under quizzes and calculators.

To test for lean/fat ratio, use a Bioelectrical Impedance Analysis (BIA) machine to evaluate precisely the risks your extra pounds actually pose. Take advantage of pharmacies that have blood pressure machines available for customer use and who sponsor cholesterol and osteoporotic screening for a nominal cost. Sometimes health fairs have numerous screenings for the price of admission.

You may find, however, that one blood sample can be used for numerous tests that don't always outrageously increase the price. Of course, you should be examining your skin and breasts regularly. Any unexplained changes may necessitate a trip to the doctor's office.

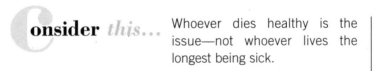

Consider *this...* Whoever dies healthy is the issue—not whoever lives the longest being sick.

CONSIDERING RISKS AND TESTS

It is never fun to discover you have a "risk" for a disease, nor is it easy to hear that some reparative action is in order. Baseline testing is likely to reveal that disease propensities exist. There is a difference between having a *risk* for a disease and having the disease itself, however. Differentiation between the two is important.

The actual danger you face and what you decide to do is equivalent to putting a rather challenging puzzle together. Test results, family history, personal health, philosophy about wellness and available financial and medical resources must all fit together. Choosing to improve overall health by stopping smoking, losing weight, eating nutritiously, drinking plenty of water, exercising your mind and body daily and working on a life in balance will not cause harm.

In contrast, the decision to take a prescribed drug or an herbal remedy because you *think* it might be protective could be harmful. Before taking anything, be aware of the risk/benefit profile. Think critically about the trade-off of drug therapy initiated concerning the risk rather than as treatment for disease. Don't forget the lesson learned from HRT!

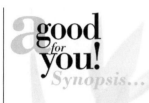

a **good** *for* **you!** *Synopsis...*

It is frustrating to have a doctor tell you your tests "prove" nothing is wrong when you feel awful. Tests that measure disease, not function, are apt to be the problem. Make sure you and your doctor look at the complete picture.

Here are some guidelines to follow when determining your current health:

1. Do not start a health program without gathering as much relevant information as you can muster and afford.

2. There is no way you can guess the true condition of your health.

3. There are clues to your health status derived from an honest look in the mirror and a little soul-searching about your self-care.

4. Always consider the risk/benefit profile of any intervention you take for risk reduction or treatment.

9

talking to your doctor

L ife is what happens after you plan" is a pithy statement I'm frequently reminded of by one of my friends. The radio host Garrison Keiller expresses the desire for perfection in his essays on life at Lake Wobegon, where "all the women are good looking and the children above average." We have the same idealized fantasies about our health. We live at "Lake Denial" where, with some exceptions, most of us are genuinely surprised and disappointed to find that our bodies somehow fail us, or are likely to.

There have been two times in my life when health issues required a complete reevaluation of my world. The first was during my pregnancy with my son. At the time, I was in near-peak physical condition. I was twenty-six years old—in my mind the perfect candidate for the perfect pregnancy, followed by the perfect child. Instead I had a very difficult time becoming pregnant and at barely four months found myself bedridden for the remainder of the pregnancy. The spinal anesthesia I refused at delivery, but got anyway, gave me a horrendous headache accompanied by severe nausea that lasted for over a week. And while my son was perfect, his gastrointestinal tract wasn't, so we spent our first weeks together crying together.

The second time I was forced to face my preconceived notions of how my life would unfold and my generalized belief that, if no longer in "peak" condition, at least my husband and I were living a healthy lifestyle, was the event of his heart attack. "How could this happen?" we asked no one in particular. There were people with far greater risk factors who were still out there having their double caramel frappaccinos, while we nursed him back to health.

There are no guarantees that anything we do will keep us from tragic health events—but that is no excuse not to try. What we don't want to do is become so obsessed with worry and fear over doing "everything" right that we make ourselves sick—or very hard to be around!

A crucial step in bringing the fantasy view of yourself as a healthy person, impervious to a major health crisis, in line with the reality of living in a world of bad bugs, poor diets, mutated genes and bodies that wear out is establishing a relationship with a health practitioner who brings a little practical reality into the scenario. Even those of us in the health professions need a health partner, a coach, if you will, who can give us pep talks when we need them, instruct us and pat us on the back when we have done well.

Sometimes finding just the right person or group of people is the hardest part of getting or staying well. In truth, you can plan on never finding him or her. You see, doctors and other health practitioners have a serious flaw—they are as human as the rest of us. The closest we can come is someone who cares, listens, communicates clearly and who admits to not knowing everything, but is knowledgeable. With such a beginning the battle is half won. Chances are, as you saw in chapter three with BMW, you are going to have to make the doctor you want and need. A little nudge here, a little push there, and you have it—a health partner.

TALKING TO THE BIG GUY OR GAL

No doubt whatever role you find yourself in at this stage of life, you have competently raised children, run an office, organized a household, painted great pictures or done similar things to "all of the above." Despite your level of confidence or competence, chances are that when you must confront your doctor, you become something just short of a wimp. It is hard to talk to an authority figure, especially one that wears a white coat, speaks "medicalese" and has had a closer look at your bottom than anyone since your mother.

Were you *wondering*? According to an NIH study, you have twenty-three seconds to set the agenda before the doctor sets it for you.[1]

Acknowledging that almost everyone finds such communication diffi-cult, this chapter will give you some suggestions for getting what you need out of your visit with a doctor. I must warn you that it requires some effort on your part. You must endeavor to learn how your body works and be aware of new discoveries that appear to roll in faster than a Nascar. However, if you want to ensure a functional view of your body and decrease the chance of a "pill for an ill" that could bring the possibility of potential risks that outweigh the benefits—read on.

GETTING WHAT YOU WANT (AND NEED) FROM A VISIT TO THE DOCTOR

"Carol, I am telling you, you are menopausal and you must take HRT," Dr. Divine insisted.

"But Doctor, my aunts all had breast cancer; I'm handling my menopause symptoms. I don't want to take hormones," Carol protested.

"Listen, I'm the doctor here, and I say you need them—either take my advice or get out of my office," was the red-faced, terse reply.

Carol gathered her jacket, picked up her purse and made her way to the door. "I'll be requesting that my medical records be sent elsewhere," she added sweetly, closing the door behind her.

I wish I could say that such a scenario never really happened, but it has, probably more times than I can imagine. Carol was enough of a critical thinker to recognize that the advice she was given was problematic and that she was being treated like a child instead of the professional, intelligent and rational woman she was. She took a deep breath and left the office because she wasn't getting what she was paying for. She wanted her doctor's opinion, but she also needed to be heard and have her point of view respectfully discussed. Have you noticed that you don't always have to have your way if you feel you have been heard?

When it comes to your health, each conversation you have with a health professional can have an outcome that can change the direction of your life. In my husband's case, the appearance of good health belied some much-skewed cholesterol levels. As we reviewed years of laboratory reports, we noted hand-written notes commending him and telling him to "keep up the good work," when what they should have done was set off alarms. While it was easy to wonder what the doctor was thinking, as responsible people we have to ask as well, "Where were we?"

Obviously, we weren't paying attention, and we selectively heard the parts we liked. A serious conversation along the way might have prevented a near-fatal heart attack, maybe not. However, there is always the chance that one conversation can change the course of your life. A missed diagnosis, an overlooked warning sign, a medication given that failed to acknowledge your size, unique metabolism or some other compounding drug you were taking can have disastrous results. Equally disastrous are the unasked questions, the misunderstood directions and the failure to comply for a myriad of unquestioned reasons.

> **T**hink about *it* ... While many are afraid of "real," it is the unreal conversation that should scare us to death.
> —SUSAN SCOTT[2]

Author Susan Scott in her book *Fierce Conversations* points out that a "conversation is the relationship."[3] The relationship deteriorates as a result of the conversations it avoids. While the nature of the relationship we have with a professional sometimes leaves us feeling humble, we must remember that we are in charge. It is our dollars that are paying for those crummy little paper robes and the advice and attention we need.

In other words, it is legitimate for you to expect something in return for your fee and a "meeting of the minds" to ensure you are on the same team. If you know you can be braver with someone to back you up, bring him or her along, or bring sixteen "hims" and "hers" along—whatever it takes to enable you to speak up, ask the questions that need asking and get done what needs to be done.

You can help out by making sure you have prepared a health history, which includes knowing as much about your family's health as possible. Share the condition of your emotional health, or let the limits of what you are willing to share be known. Include medications you are on along with their dosage, and don't exclude nutritional supplements or natural medicines. I have a friend who has a written history of every doctor's visit and lab report he has had for the last eight years. Maybe such diligence is not for you, but, minimally, how hard is it to create a file for "medical reports" in which information such as dates of visits, tests, medication and laboratory reports can be kept?

Do some reflective thinking about how you have handled yourself the last few visits to a medical professional. How did you react if you felt scared? What did you do if the conversation did not go well? When you didn't understand, did you speak up? Did you try to control the situation and tell the doctor what you needed without listening in return? Were your questions and comments clear and to the point, or were they vague references to "not feeling well"? Did you ask questions? If something you said came out wrong, were you able to say, "I need to restate what I just said; it didn't come out right, and I want to be sure you hear what I am trying to say." If you were misheard, were you able to say, "I'm hearing that you heard me say…but I was really saying…"?

Preparing yourself

Once you realize your strengths and weaknesses conversationally, maximize the chance for a good conversation by spending some time specifically preparing for your visit. Besides helping you clarify what you want to accomplish, the time spent in organization will result in greater quality time once you are in the office. Doctors are under tremendous pressure to get patients in and on their way. The more succinct you can be, the more time there will be for discussion. Should you find the conversation is more complex and time-consuming than you thought it would be, reschedule for continuation if your physician is pressed for time. If you know you need additional time in advance, make that clear to the scheduling nurse and insist on a longer appointment.

The following is adapted from *Fierce Conversations*.[4] You will find the suggestions helpful in preparing for a discussion with your medical practitioner.

1. *Be clear and concise about what the issue is:* "Doctor, I'm here today because I need to know whether to stay on HRT or discontinue its use."

2. *Know why it is important:* "I am concerned about my risk for breast cancer, but tests have indicated that I have lost bone to the point that I am in danger of having a fracture."

3. *What would be an ideal outcome:* "I would like to get off HRT, but I don't want to put myself at greater risk for osteoporosis."

4. *Share the background:* "My grandmother broke her hip and never again walked unaided. I am a very busy and active person. I have my own business and three grandchildren I adore. It is important to me to stay active."

5. *What has been done:* "I have been on HRT for five years and have increased my bone strength. I participate in a walking group and have made sure I am taking a top-quality calcium product."

6. *This is what I need:* "I need you to advise me on my individual risk for breast cancer and what options are available should I discontinue HRT. Also, if I stop HRT, I need to know how to do that."

When things go wrong

Let's say that despite your good intentions and preplanning, the conversation does not go well. Or, just as nerve wracking, you aren't sure what the doctor is thinking. What are you to do then?[5] If you have carefully clarified your end of the conversation, it is legitimate to state, "If you see my concerns differently, I would like to hear what you have to say."

Or, simply, what is your perspective? Perhaps you might add, "I've told you my concern. Could you share with me how you see it from your side? Then let me react to your thinking and see what you think." If being diplomatic is your thing, try something like: "I feel this is the right course for me; what might I be missing?"

While Carol undoubtedly did the best thing in response to Dr. Divine's arrogance, she could have decided to give him another chance by saying something like, "I admit I see the issue very differently, but before I jump to conclusions, tell me what you have seen or heard that leads you to see it the way you do" or, "I feel I am between the proverbial rock and a hard place; I want to talk openly but I am afraid I have (will) upset you." Should Dr. Divine share his reasoning, and it is lacking in logic and doesn't pass the critical thinking criteria, Carol could then ask, "Can you help me understand how you came up with that?" or, "Why do you think that is so?"

How do you know the visit was a success?

"You are effective to the extent that there is a match between your intentions and your outcomes."[6]

Why should you bother taking the time to organize the goals of your visit and practice techniques of keeping communication lines open? Your goal is to create an atmosphere in which your concerns can be discussed in a milieu of trust and respect in order for you to learn how to maintain your optimal state of wellness and be affirmed in your efforts.

Helping yourself to "seconds"

It may surprise you to learn that fewer than one in four Americans facing life-threatening illnesses get a second opinion.[7] It is true that most second opinions confirm the first, but for the few who have a diagnosis changed, medication adjusted or who choose a different chemotherapy path, it can be life changing. Without an outside opinion, there is little likelihood that a new path will be decided upon or a misdiagnosis corrected. If the medical issue you are dealing with is rare or atypical—a young woman with heart disease, a man with a breast lump, for instance—there is even more reason to seek additional evaluation.

Sometimes the second opinion takes the form of a second look at laboratory results. Johns Hopkins University Medical Institutions examined six thousand pathology reports over twenty-one months and found only 1.4 percent errors. But when the information was broken down, it was discovered that errors occur more frequently with some diagnoses than they do with others. The rate of error increased to 5.1 percent with cancers of the female reproductive tract, and for cancers of membranes that line the body cavities, such as stomach cancer, the rate jumped to 9.5 percent. Liver biopsy samples reviewed at the University of Miami School of Medicine revealed that 28 percent required a change in both diagnosis and treatment.[8] While not exactly a second opinion, there are laws in forty-two states and the District of Columbia that give patients the right to an independent review in appealing a treatment decision by their HMO or managed care plan. Your insurance company decides who pays for a consultation, but often the option is there if you insist. Despite the trust and confidence you have in your physician, it is always wise to be resolute about the need for a second opinion in the case of complex, life-threatening diseases or when a reasonable treatment time has not resulted in improvement. The complexity of modern medicine and technology makes it essential. You and your doctor may need highly technical advice only available from research centers.

The major reason given for not asking for a second opinion is fear of offending the doctor. A good physician will welcome the affirmation of his or her plan of treatment and the confidence and commitment it gives you, the patient, that the road you are on is leading where it is supposed to lead.

WHY WE DO WHAT WE DO

Most of us do not know why we do what we do regarding medical choices. Perhaps we have always done what our parents modeled or insisted upon or whatever our doctors told us to do. As we have grown older, other influences have weighed in: our friends, television and magazines, even the clerk at the health food store. Choosing to go to a natural practitioner is no guarantee that we still might not go blindly into the night, not questioning.

If you have a problem defining to yourself your relationship with your doctor, remember that no one knows your body, your feelings, your needs better than you. The question is, "Do you act like you do?" If not, why not?

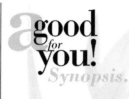

1. Are you able to have a conversation with your doctor? Are you easily intimidated by authority? Can you take someone with you?

2. Where does most of your medical information come from? Friends? Doctors? Health food clerks? Reading? Internet? News?

3. What process do you use for deciding if you should adopt a health practice? Why, for instance, do you take vitamins (or not)?

4. How do you deal with a crisis in your life? Are you a minimizer? Do you panic?

5. What is your typical response when you are suffering?

10

the first leg: nutrition

Somewhere in each of our homes, currently or back in the days when bookshelves were bricks and boards, there is a three-legged table. You know what I'm talking about—the kind made of the cheapest material but meant to be covered by just the right cloth that skims the floor and transforms it into something even Martha Stewart could love. Remember the time it collapsed right in the middle of serving tea to Mrs. Judg-u-now? Or, perhaps it still stands in the guest bedroom, a bit catawampus, but out of the way. Keep its image in mind because there is no better metaphor for a health foundation.

When the legs are not screwed on correctly or become loose, the table becomes very unbalanced. No one in their right mind actually places anything they value on its top without insuring that the legs are solidly screwed and maybe even glued into position. Now think of that three-legged table as representative of your health. The legs symbolize your *nutrition, exercise and stress management.* Each "leg" is essential. When any one is unstable, the foundation for your health is a catastrophe waiting to happen.

So, before we begin to make suggestions for the specifics of care for symptoms of menopause or other age-related concerns, take a minute and consider the condition of your health "table." If you are like two-thirds of Americans, you are carrying extra weight and are making too many stops at fast-food places. As for exercise, is it possible that getting up and down from the table is a full day's activity? And, although you may no longer be chewing your nails, is stress eating you up?

In the rest of this chapter, we will consider the first leg, *nutrition.* What goes in eventually comes out, but an incredible number of things happen in between. You may think the hamburger you ate for lunch is insignificant, but it is not treated as insignificant by your gastrointestinal tract, also known as your "gut." The gut is selective and protective. It even rebels. Can you describe a rebellious gut?

The goal here is not to give you a methodical eating plan that works for Lyra or me, but to help you understand that through paying attention to your body's response to food you will uncover your unique nutritional requirements. You should be able to discern foods that rebel because they make you tired or "sluggish," they make your nose run or clog your sinuses, and they cause bloating, gas, diarrhea or constipation. Sometimes the rebellion is immediate, but there could be as much as a twenty-four- to thirty-six-hour delay.

Feed your troops (body systems and individual cells) what they need, and the rebellion is not only squelched, but also "in-fighting," where one division steals from another to get what it needs to survive another day, will cease. The result? Peace. In a peaceful "gut" environment, energy previously used on the battlefront is unrestricted and redirected in ways that heal and give you a renewed vitality. Eliminating skirmishes reduces the chance of debilitating illnesses, improves the odds of controlling your weight and sets up a line of defense against outside invaders. If you are sick and tired of being sick and tired, declare a truce between you and your gut; consider what you eat.

something *to* *think about*

Die-hard vegetarians continue to rail against dietary fat and emulate Chinese peasants. Born-again carnivores blame the White Devil (a.k.a. bread) and force themselves to go on all-meat diets in hopes of incinerating their belly fat. Ordinary civilians throw up their hands and consume whatever is convenient— which is to say Krispy Kremes and Coke.[1]

How do you do that? Start with careful observation of your unique food metabolism. Second, consider balance. If your diet is highly restrictive and unbalanced in any direction, it is not right for you. Finally, if you feel deprived, you are not eating well. Healthy eating is not synonymous with being "tasteless."

Hopefully, you do not consider the benefits of nutritious food as limited to a *source of fuel*. Let's switch our analogy from the battlefield to your car. It needs to have oil changes and tune-ups in addition to gas to keep it in top condition. While food is a source of fuel, it also provides the fine-tuning, cleaning-out, outright adjustment and other minutia of maintenance that keep the mechanism running. Your body gets a tune-up after every meal. If what you ate was metabolically sound for your unique body and the state of your health, like a well-maintained car, you will run well and last longer.

You are your own mechanic. Are you a good one? You do not have to be on a macrobiotic diet, never eat another chocolate chip cookie or get a degree in nutrition to do a stellar job. Mostly, you need to use common sense. A personalized mechanic's manual with your name on it exists in the form of your genes and includes the particular biochemical reactions that best maximize your health. More pages are added to your mechanic's manual as scientists pinpoint the "nutrigenomics" that make all of us tick.

Bottom line, every new page of your personal manual reinforces that what you eat matters. A dramatic confirmation was reported in a television news story of a young mother who, on a lark, sent in the DNA swab kit she received following delivery of her baby girl. The company that had included it, along with the other take-home gifts for new mothers, tested for a number of genetic disorders. This seemingly healthy baby girl had a genetic mutation involving a defective protein enzyme that would have taken her life by age ten had it not been discovered. The remedy to ensure a healthy and long life was strictly nutritional.

Never lose sight of the fact that although we all love the social and sharing aspects of eating, food remains the most powerful *medicine* you take. And for those of you with a few extra pounds, it isn't true that you need sugar to help the medicine go down. Fresh, full-flavored food close to the source is satisfying. Modern technology is supplying the explanation for the ancient adage that "you are what you eat."

IS EATING THERAPEUTICALLY AS BAD AS IT SOUNDS?

With nutritional advice coming from every direction, who or what can you trust? After all, for the last ten years Americans have adopted the government's guidelines and have become fatter than ever.

Thanks to Dr. Walter Willett and his colleagues at the Harvard School of Public Health, more trustworthy advice is available. Gleaning everything that is known about the relationship between what a person eats and the diseases they have (or do not have) from large studies such as the Nurses' Health Study, the Physicians' Health Study and the Health Professionals' Follow-Up Study, they introduced the Healthy Eating Pyramid.[2] The recommendations are meant to be adopted as a lifetime eating plan, not a diet. This Healthy Eating Pyramid notes distinctions within food groups. Our government's recommended pyramid declared that all fat was bad and all carbohydrates good. By contrast, Dr. Willett points out that differences in fat make certain versions of it essential and that white, processed types of carbohydrates are likely to make us fat, whereas whole-grain versions are not only more nutritious but aren't as quick to pack on pounds.

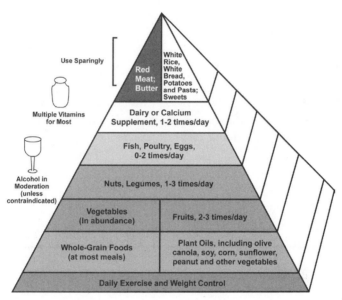

From Walter C. Willett, M.D., *Eat, Drink, and Be Healthy* (New York: Simon and Schuster, 2001). Used with permission.

The Healthy Eating Pyramid's foundation is exercise and weight control. The base of the pyramid consists of whole-grain foods, vegetable oils, and fruits and vegetables. At the top with the recommendation "use sparingly," which means occasionally and in approximately 3-ounce portions, is red meat from which absorbable iron, magnesium and zinc can be obtained. Refined grains such as white bread and white rice are also in the limited category.

While most people worry about the fat content in nuts, responding to data that "nut-eaters" are thinner than people with a tendency to be overweight, along with the fact that nuts contain healthful nutrients, nuts and legumes (beans and peas) are placed in their own category in the pyramid. These foods have the added advantage of helping people feel full.

Protein sources, previously lumped together, are now acknowledged to differ in their therapeutic diet value—fish, shellfish, poultry and eggs being preferable to cheeses, other dairy products and other meats. Studies have shown that lecithin in eggs blocks absorption of cholesterol, which explains why they are once again recommended. The option exists to obtain necessary calcium from a supplement or dairy product. Alcohol in moderation and a multivitamin are a surprise addition for many.

While no schematic gives a complete picture, the concept is based on sound nutritional science, and its implementation is feasible. It provides a starting point from which you can make your individual adjustments. While the numbers of servings are recommended, the size of the servings is best calculated with your eyes. Your palm is a good gauge for the size of your protein source. Allocate a handful of carbohydrates like potatoes, rice or pasta, or substitute whole-grain bread or dessert for this serving if you are trying to lose weight and would rather have a "treat," and allow yourself plenty of vegetables and salad. Fruit makes a healthy dessert.

antioxidant phytochemicals in foods

CLASS	FOOD SOURCE
TERPENES Carotenoids Lycopene Lutein and zeaxanthin Capsaicin	Carrot, yam, apricot, yellow tomato, red grapefruit, spinach, kale, turnip greens, red chili peppers
PHENOLS Anthocyanins Anthoxanthins Betacyanin Catechins Flavonols and proanthocyani- dins Flavonoids Lignans Resveratrol	Concord grapes, eggplant, cauliflower, potato, beets, green and black tea, grape seeds, citrus fruits, berries, peppers, flaxseed, wheat berry, barley, grape skin
ORGANIC ACIDS Ellagic acid Glyceritinic acid	Strawberries, grapes, apples, licorice root

low-glycemic carbohydrate choices

Fruits	Apples, apricots, cherries, grapefruit, oranges, peaches, plums
Vegetables	Artichoke, asparagus, broccoli, cauliflower, green beans, lettuce/greens
Grains	Oatmeal, rye, wild rice (brown or basmati), whole-grain products
Legumes	Black beans, chick peas, kidney beans, lentils
Starches	Sweet potatoes, whole-grain pasta, yams

It is important that you understand that all foods in a category do not have the same effect on the body. Carbohydrates, found in many foods, but particularly abundant in grains and rice, metabolize into sugar at different rates. Those that waste no time, like a big chocolate chip cookie, are called *high-glycemic* carbohydrates. Those that take their time, like vegetables, are categorized as *low-glycemic* carbohydrates. Why does it matter?

Sugar in the bloodstream sends a signal to the pancreas to release the hormone insulin. When there is a lot of sugar, insulin levels become very high. Insulin has a big job to do and can choose to do it in several ways; the bottom line is that it must reduce the sugar (glucose) in the bloodstream. Some glucose is used by the cells as fuel for energy production, but insulin also sees to it that any excess glucose is stored as a fat cell for future use. After a large meal or a high-glycemic snack, insulin becomes particularly plentiful and efficient and quickly reduces blood sugar—so much, in fact, that it leaves you in short supply.

Sensing you now don't have enough sugar to function properly (you are light-headed and hungry), your body goes into alarm mode telling you to search for something to eat, preferably something you instinctively know will give you a fast boost—something sweet. You down a doughnut, insulin again pours into your system, and this feast or famine cycle is repeated again and again. Every insulin cycle squirrels away a few more fat cells in preparation for the day you can't find a snack. The result for all but a lucky 25 percent of the population, whose carbohydrate intake has little effect on their metabolism, is weight gain, especially for another 25 percent who appear very sensitive to weight gain after eating carbohydrates.

The more processed the food, the more quickly it is digested—a doughnut versus a slice of Irish brown bread, for example. Select fruit over fruit juices or soft drinks. Eat pasta slightly undercooked—like the Italians. Add vinegar or lemon juice to carbohydrate foods; the acid slows their rate of absorption about 30 percent. Opt for sourdough or grainy bread—bagels can't wait to become sugar. Choose slow-cooked oatmeal and "all bran" over processed cereals.

Some people crave carbohydrates because of their ability to improve mood. Carbohydrates increase the production of serotonin. That piece of chocolate cake works like a natural tranquilizer or antidepressant, but with the side effect of extra fat. The urge to grab a "goodie" to allay fear, anxiety or sadness isn't just lack of will power; it has biological roots.

Falling levels of estrogen lower insulin secretion and decrease insulin sensitivity, a partial explanation for why you tend to gain weight at midlife. Progesterone increases insulin secretion and insulin resistance, offering a partial explanation for carbohydrate cravings before a monthly period. To avoid the carbohydrate roller coaster, blood sugar levels must be maintained throughout the day. You can do this by eating frequent smaller meals and being careful in your selection of carbohydrates, which must be balanced by proper portions of protein and fat to slow absorption and help you feel full. A diet high in fiber (beans, bran, brown rice and vegetables like broccoli, asparagus and spinach) helps control blood sugar while keeping you feeling full. Note: A quick way to put on a few pounds is to skip breakfast.

A closer look at fats

Saturated fats are mostly animal fats that are solid at room temperature. Plant-based versions include liquid coconut, palm and palm kernel oil. Saturated fat tells the liver to make artery-clogging LDL cholesterol. When we eat too much, they increase the risk of heart disease and cancer, among other health problems. Unsaturated fats are usually liquid and either polyunsaturated (safflower, corn, soybean, fish) or monounsaturated (olive, sesame and canola oils, almonds, avocado). Monounsaturated fats like olive oil lower LDL and increase HDL, protecting against heart disease and benefiting the body in a number of other ways.

something
to think about

Good guy fats include cold-water fish (salmon, mackerel, tuna, herring, crab, etc.), avocados, raw nuts, nut butters, seeds, olive oil, canola, flaxseed, sunflower and pumpkinseed.

Essential fatty acids (EFA), including omega-3, are essential because the body can't make them; they must come from food or supplements. Fish oils, fish, flax, borage, black currant and primrose oil, sunflower and pumpkinseeds are wonderful sources. They boost energy, reduce heart disease and pain from arthritis. EFAs heighten immunity. Signs of depletion include fatigue, lack of endurance, dry skin and hair and frequent colds.

Hydrogenated vegetable oils (transfatty acids) have recently been declared unsafe at any level. Transfatty acids are used in foods to help them maintain taste and last while they sit on a shelf for an indefinite amount of time. Like saturated fats they lower healthy cholesterol, HDL, and are linked to cancer and diabetes. You won't find them listed on any product you buy, but that is to change soon. Your clue is a label that includes "partially hydrogenated oils," including those claiming to be "fat" free or to have "no cholesterol."

Where does chocolate fit?

Good chocolate is rich in antioxidant flavonoids called flavanols (procyanidins, epicatechins, catechins), known to lower the risk of heart disease, lung cancer, asthma and diabetes. Some studies have shown benefits to HDL and LDL ratios, and for lowering clotting and keeping arteries flexible. This is good news for those of you who love chocolate—as long as you are willing to buy the best. One ounce of high-quality, very special chocolate has double the antioxidant punch of red wine or other dark chocolates.

And what about alcohol?

While no one would suggest anyone who doesn't drink should start, alcohol in moderation (one drink per day) has been shown to be protective against heart disease. When the *moderate* line is ignored, the effect on health can be very negative. Of most concern is the 41 percent increase in breast cancer in women with two to five drinks per day (9 percent in women with less than one drink per day).[3] Because women have more fatty tissue than men, which contains less water than muscle, there is less body water available to dilute alcohol. Additionally, women metabolize alcohol differently. The key gastric enzyme that degrades alcohol is lower in women than in men, allowing more alcohol to pass through the stomach and enter the blood. To make matters worse, women are more vulnerable to liver disease, and if they have an alcohol problem, they are more likely to develop a quickly deteriorating alcoholic hepatitis and cirrhosis of the liver. They are also more susceptible to alcohol-related cardiomyopathy, a weakening of the heart muscle.

Tea...can it save your life?

Despite the fact that Americans love their coffee, after water, tea is the most consumed drink in the world. Asian cultures have recognized a medicinal component for generations. Tea is rich in antioxidants (polyphenols and flavonoids), and research has verified its cancer-protectiveness and its ability to lower the risk of heart disease.[4] However, most people drink tea because it tastes good and relaxes them. The relaxation effect is due to a neurologically active amino acid, L-theanine, found almost exclusively in tea plants. (Note: High-grade Matcha green tea, Gyokuro and Sencha green teas and Ceylon Pekoe, Sri Lanka, Darjeeling and Earl Grey black teas are likely to have higher L-theanine levels.) This ingredient explains why tea, with its higher caffeine content than coffee, does not produce the same "wired" effect. Both green tea and black tea appear protective if consumed on a regular basis. These teas are not the same as herbal teas, which may have their own medicinal use.

The healthy pyramid around the world

Asian and Mediterranean diets have been touted as healthier than the American diet. It is a common experience to have disease profiles change for the worse when people adopt a Western diet. The value of both the Asian and Mediterranean diets, which are really quite different, is an emphasis on vegetables and small amounts of protein, particularly fish. It has been observed that the Chinese have very long life spans, except for the very poor. A Japanese diet is particularly healthy because it includes more fish.

something *to think about*

High-quality protein choices include fish, chicken and turkey, tofu and tempeh, egg and egg whites, low-fat cottage cheese.

The Mediterranean diet includes nuts, fish, plenty of fresh vegetables, salads, beans, olive oil and wine. The food is minimally processed, and fresh fruit often serves as dessert. Olive oil is the main source of fat. Cheese and yogurt may be consumed daily but in small amounts; red meat may be consumed rarely. It is a diet high in omega-3 fatty acids obtained through fish, walnuts and green leafy vegetables. The carbohydrates are not from Krispy Kreme.

Because the Mediterranean diet is very satisfying, studies of weight loss using a moderate-fat Mediterranean-style diet as compared to a low-fat diet have resulted in better long-term participation and adherence and greater loss of weight. Most people experience it as delicious, hearty and healthy.[5] It is a diet close to the one that the French consume.

A word about organics

There is a general consensus among the scientific community that toxic pollutants are increasing at an astounding rate. Our bodies are working overtime to deal with substances they have never faced before or in amounts they were never meant to handle. It is reasonable to think in terms of how one might reduce the toxic load with which your body must contend. While many exposures are out of our hands, we have a degree of control when we choose organic food.

There are many reasons for developing a small garden, beyond harvesting some of your own pesticide-free food and herbs; it can be emotionally satisfying and calming. Aside from that, most communities have farmer's markets or grocery stores where organic products are sold. Why would you bother? Food products without added chemicals put less stress on your body's detoxification processes and reduce the chance of triggering metabolic changes that can lead to poor health, including cancer. They also provide more nutrients (60 percent more flavonoids in corn grown without chemicals).

Until October 2002, organic labeling meant very little. Currently the United States Department of Agriculture (USDA) has established the following guidelines: An organic label means that 95 percent of the ingredients must be organic, and products with 70–94 percent organic ingredients can be labeled "made with organic ingredients." If fewer than 70 percent of the ingredients are organic, the product cannot be labeled organic, but may list the organic ingredients.

Don't forget the obvious

Water is an essential part of good health, making up 70 percent of body weight. Diets that promise quick weight losses are really eliminating water or muscle, since only one or two pounds of fat cells can be lost per week. When you are in short supply of water, a hormone is released to retain water and sodium.

WHY WE HAVE BECOME ONE OF THE
FATTEST NATIONS IN THE WORLD

The National Institutes of Health and the U.S. Surgeon General declare "the top ten causes of death due to disease are attributable to health risks associated with excess body fat." The NIH states, "Obesity is a leading cause of heart disease, hypertension, stroke, diabetes and even cancer."[6]

Age has something to do with it. After age thirty, the rate at which we break down our food and the efficiency with which we utilize or store it begin to slow down—1 percent a year. As a result of a creeping metabolism and the fact that we tend to begin creeping through our exercise routines, weight stealthily increases unless the simple decision is made to eat less and exercise more.

Part of the problem is that we eat *the wrong kinds of food*. Our penchant for "low-fat" products and "white" foods hasn't kept us thin.

Far from color and the garden, they are "life-less" high-glycemic options with little nutritional value and a negative metabolic effect. The tendency toward highly processed foods with shelf lives that rival Methuselah has contributed greatly to the American increase in weight and food-related diseases. As a result, the "standard American diet" is only half-jokingly referred to as "SAD." We know it is possible to eat well and stay slim because the French do it. They are the most slender of all Europeans.

---

something *to think about*

Our recommendation is to begin eating in a therapeutically nutritional way while focusing on increasing your fitness and making sure you do not gain more weight.

We have also outgrown our breeches because we eat *too much*. Portions in restaurants have grown to gargantuan sizes. A 3-ounce serving of meat is lost in the shadow of the 8-, 12- or 16-ounce steak. One pasta serving is enough for a week and is now brought to you on a 12-inch plate. Servings of soft drinks have topped 64 ounces, ten times the original Coke bottle.

These proportions, you note, are a far cry from what is recommended by the Healthy Food Pyramid. Some wit has suggested that our food is not served, it is shoveled. Recently, nutritionists at Pennsylvania State University studied the "psychology of food portions." Whether study participants served themselves or had food given to them in measured amounts, people inevitably ate more when they had a larger portion. Interestingly, eating the larger portions did not make them feel more full than when they ate smaller portions, and less than half noticed any difference in portion size when they were served.[7] The bad news is that we tend to eat what we are served; the good news is that smaller portions leave us satisfied.

BACK TO—WHAT NEXT?

Good for You! is not about to give you yet another diet. Here again you must think critically about what is going to work long term for you. *Our recommendation is to begin eating in a therapeutically nutritional way while focusing on increasing your fitness and making sure you do not gain more weight.* Just that much would have a positive impact on your health. If you truly believe that food is potent medicine, you owe it to yourself to insure the correct prescription. Once you are eating well for your health and body, and feeling more fit, you may find yourself more motivated to take extra steps to lose weight.

To lose weight permanently or to maintain your weight, you must change your pattern of eating. It must become your lifestyle instead of a grueling period of time when you deny yourself. Even small changes can make a difference: eliminating sugar in coffee, getting rid of soft drinks and eating only one cookie. A reduction of as little as one hundred calories a day, especially when combined with just fifteen minutes of extra exercise per day, is enough to prevent weight gain for most people.[8] You can do that.

THINKING ABOUT DIETING DIFFERENTLY

Scientists used to believe that once you celebrated your sixtieth birthday, you could also celebrate that your weight problems were over. But the government's Centers for Disease Control and Prevention studies have put that myth to bed. Americans aged sixty to seventy-four years old are gaining weight faster than any other age group. While it is true that your risk of dying sooner is only slightly higher if you are obese compared to your same-age slim friend, that is only part of the story. The rest of the story is quality of life. The closer you are to your ideal weight, the greater your energy, mobility and likelihood of independence will be as you age.

A CONSIDERATION YOU MUST NOT OVERLOOK

Much of what is considered "aging" is loss of muscle. Muscle loss occurs naturally and is harder to maintain as we get older. As we become weaker and less active, further loss is escalated. You gain weight because muscle burns more calories than fat, and with the loss of muscle, your fat-burning machine is missing. Therefore, building and maintaining muscle is crucial to maintaining and losing weight.

As we have mentioned, quick weight loss can be due to breaking down muscle rather than fat. You look trim, but the ratio of muscle to body fat has shifted, and keeping weight off becomes increasingly difficult. Muscles are also a source of protein; loss of protein in muscles means loss of function elsewhere. If you happen to become ill, you have fewer muscle cells for the manufacture of antibodies, wound healing and white blood cell production.

something
***to* think about**

Maintaining muscle strength fights aging, illness and weight gain simultaneously.

Muscle mass can also be lost as a result of insulin resistance, which is tied to gaining weight and to immune factors. Maintaining muscle strength fights aging, illness and weight gain simultaneously.

How do you find out what your body composition is?

Another way of asking this is, "How much of my body is lean mass, and how much is fat?" Your doctor, chiropractor, personal trainer or nutritionist is apt to have a Bioelectrical Impedance Analysis (BIA) machine that determines your body composition. This is different from the body mass index, which measures the likelihood of obesity. (See chapter eight.)

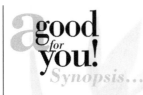

Facing the bottom line:

1. What keeps you from adopting a diet of unprocessed, organic, well-balanced foods?

2. What motivates you when you do make healthy choices?

3. Do you categorize foods as "good" or "bad" based on principles of dieting instead of "healthy" and "unhealthy"?

4. Can you begin to monitor your portions? Why or why not?

5. What is your excuse for not eating smaller, more frequent "meals"?

6. If you make one small step toward a healthier diet, what will it be?

11

the second and third legs: exercise and stress management

In deference to the KISS (Keep It Simple, Stupid) philosophy, there is one thing to be remembered—exercise can't be beat for improving your health. The truth is, living a long time subjects you to normal wear and tear. Allowing your body to become weak is a major factor in aging; a weak body is often *confused* with aging. No wonder that by age seventy-five, 66 percent of women can't lift objects heavier than ten pounds.

A MIRACLE DRUG

As the mechanic of your body, you recognize that, like your car, all the bells, whistles and fluids are going to work better if you get it out of the garage regularly and take it for a spin. Exercise is a miracle drug you can afford. Unless you insist on fancy outfits and an expensive gym membership, it costs little more than a good pair of walking shoes. While anything that gets you moving is good, walking can have a profound effect on your health.

It will increase your metabolic rate so that even on the days you spend reading a book, you will burn more calories. Your body composition will change as you build muscle, which positively affects insulin and blood sugar control, lowering your risk for cardiovascular and other diseases. Exercise enables you to sleep better but have more energy when you want to be active. Equally important, since your brain cell functioning improves—you will remember what you did!

Other than a bug bite or a sprained ankle, there is no down side. Yet, it is estimated that one in four Americans lead a completely sedentary life. If that is true for you, make sure you have a checkup before you start any exercise program.

Goal: long term

When you do start, your goal is long term; don't decide to attend six classes a week or jog five miles—start slowly. Build up to at least thirty minutes on most days, including warming up, walking and cooling down. That is enough to be beneficial. How fast should you go? Just three to three and one-half miles per hour, or one mile in fifteen or twenty minutes is fine. If you like gadgets, you can purchase a pedometer (a device that measures the distance you walk) and make sure you get at least ten thousand steps total throughout each day—about five miles. If you add two thousand more steps (about a mile) you will prevent weight gain, according to researchers at the University of Colorado.[1]

something
to think about

Exercise is a miracle drug you can afford.

Add more steps by losing your television remote control one day a week, walk through museums or galleries, or take a twirl around the local mall if the weather is inclement. Mix socializing with friends with your walk, or stride with grandkids. Get a dog; they won't take no for an answer. Set up a "beep" break with an alarm device, where you get up and walk or exercise for ten minutes at least three times per day. Stand on one foot when brushing your teeth, stretch while reaching for something in a cabinet, plié while you rinse dishes, walk while talking on the phone, and deep breathe while standing in line and at every red light.

In a study of 73,743 postmenopausal women published in September 2002 by JoAnn Manson of Brigham and Women's Hospital (affiliated with Harvard), it was found that women cut their risk of heart disease by up to 40 percent with thirty minutes of exercise, even by gardening and yard work. Thirty minutes lowered the risk of chronic diseases; sixty minutes in combination with a diet was enough to reduce weight. Breaking up your thirty minutes a day improves mood while still contributing to overall fitness. Research confirms regular physical activity is an important and potent protective factor for preventing cognitive decline and dementia in elderly persons.[2] In a study of women (aged sixty-five or older) who walked and were given memory tests over six to eight years, those who walked the most, all else being equal, had less chance of experiencing cognitive decline.[3]

Make it play

If the thought of exercise makes you nauseous, play instead. What kinds of things did you enjoy as a kid? No one ever came to your door and asked you to come out and *exercise,* but you got plenty when you went out to *play.* My current involvement with in-line skating directly relates to long-gone, care-free days at a local skating rink. Now while I'm grinning ear-to-ear with all the eleven-year-olds, I'm also bending, stretching, getting my heartbeat racing and using every muscle in my body to keep upright. Golf, on the other hand, is a new sport for me. It gets me walking, and since I need more swings than most to reach the green, I'm assured of plenty of squats and twists. Just being outside lowers my stress level and improves my mood. What did you love as a kid? Have you wanted to salsa dance? Reinstate the "play" in your life.

Another advantage of "playing" your exercise is that you are likely to get all three components of a well-rounded program: aerobics for your circulation and stamina, stretching to keep you flexible and moving about, and strengthening to counteract the normal muscle loss of aging. And play, I have discovered, is a natural sleep aid and mood elevator. No one is suggesting you do something you hate; find what suits your personality and stick to it. Any exercise is better than no exercise. The good news is that the more out-of-condition you are, the more you will benefit.

Enhancing balance

If you are past forty, you may have noticed a decline in your balance. This is why exercise programs like Tai Chi are so beneficial. Improve your balance and decrease the risk of falls—very important if your bones are thinning. Once a hip is broken, the statistics for returning to the same active life are grim. Strength training is an important component of balance because your muscles can't respond if they are too weak. Add muscle by slowly lifting weights. Begin with a weight you can lift eight to twelve times, and when that becomes easy, add more. Sometimes working with a personal trainer is helpful to get you going and to design a program that is right for you. His or her motivation (and the fact you are probably paying him or her) helps to get you into the habit. Strive for twenty minutes of weight training three times a week.

There is no other way to improve muscle mass except regular exercise. Too many women accept that becoming weak is part of aging and can be explained by changes in hormones. The fact that losing muscle tends to escalate at midlife is coincidental, not causative. While aging naturally reduces metabolism, the major reason the resting metabolic rate becomes slow is reduction in lean body mass. *The less your muscle mass, the slower your metabolism.* You must minimize muscle loss and increase muscle mass if you intend to keep active and prevent weight gain. Strength training not only increases your muscle mass and increases your metabolic rate while you are lifting those cans of peas, but also it will continue to do so for a time at an accelerated rate after the exercise session has ended.

Because the baby boomers are finding exercising to rock music no longer gives them the charge it did in the past, and because their knees have likely rebelled, kinder, gentler exercise classes have come into vogue. Yoga is enjoyed for its focus on flexibility and stretching as well as its ability to release a lifetime of stress held tightly in muscles and joints. After years of an emphasis in gyms on building up big arms and strong legs, Pilates (and yoga) have refocused attention to the torso, building up core strength to support and create flexibility in the spine through slow, controlled movements. This new approach to fitness is called "functional fitness," which means "well-rounded." Isn't that interesting, and doesn't it sound familiar? Core strength develops key muscles needed for strengthening your middle and holding you upright.

Were you *wondering*? Does exercise work if you are obese? Regular exercise, such as brisk walking, reduces body weight and fat among those overweight or obese.[4]

No pill is as good or safe as exercise is for reducing the risk of all major diseases. Give yourself a health goal as motivation for increasing your physical activity. The weight you lose by increasing your activity is much more likely to stay off. And don't ever think you are too old to begin to get into shape. Studies prove that people in their nineties can build muscle, and those who stay active postpone the development of disabilities. Tufts University found that seventy- and eighty-year-olds who did thirty minutes of moderate strength training a week built muscle—even though they ate more.[5] Now there is a plan! What is your plan going to be?

THE THIRD LEG OF YOUR HEALTH FOUNDATION TABLE: STRESS MANAGEMENT

It is well documented that 75–90 percent of all visits to primary care physicians are for stress-related complaints or disorders. While big stressors like death or losses of any kind take their toll, the most dangerous variety is the never-ending and lower-level version that literally "eats away" at you. Unremitting stress makes you sick. When stressed, your hypothalamus, pituitary and adrenal glands are called into action to shut down what is not essential to keeping you alive or helping you through a crisis. The impact of this "survival mode" is felt throughout the body.

Still, stress is not all bad. It is essential for growth and health. Stressing a muscle, for example, is the only way to build muscle mass. The surge of adrenaline before giving a speech can help you remember your lines and be lively and entertaining. The infamous "flight-or-fight" response gets you out of trouble by giving a surge of high-powered energy to jump out of the way of a speeding car.

> **Think about** *it ...* A study that looked at people who had lost weight and kept it off found they generally did one hour of moderate physical activity daily, ate five small meals or snacks, monitored their weight and almost never ate fast food.[6]

The problem with stress

The problem with stress lies in two areas. The first is the fact that most of us live a stress-filled existence. The second, that once the stress response is turned on, it doesn't take much to *keep* it on. When used continually, any machine eventually wears out and breaks. The same happens with the body. In particular, when the adrenal glands are primed to respond around the clock, they wear out, too.

While you may be able to turn down the stress response, it is unlikely you will be able to rid yourself of stress completely. The realistic choice is to learn how to handle stress well. Stressors are not always as obvious as you might think. Environmental stress includes noise or chemical exposure. Internal stress can be the end result of a nutritional deficiency such as a high-sugar and high-fat diet, being in pain or even sleeping poorly. Whatever the source, sooner or later the cumulative effect causes a break-down in the mechanism that keeps the so-called "flight-or-fight" response under control. That breakdown event can be as much of a problem as the original threat itself.

What happens when we are stressed?

It is true that some people are more susceptible to stress than others.

Apart from the drama of their lives and personal coping mechanisms, a genetic component is at work. Consider what happens to a typical midlife woman we will call Diane, who, like many women, is feeling the effects of an accumulation of life's events. Diane is forty-eight years old and perimenopausal. She lives alone fifty miles from her mother whom she visits once a week. Her father died years ago, and her mother has remained independent.

something
to think about

The realistic choice is to learn how to handle stress well.

Last week Diane received a phone call from a neighbor who found her mother wandering in the rain, dressed in her nightgown and searching for a dog that had died years before. Diane had noticed disturbing changes in her mother, but she ignored them, especially when her brother, who visited once every few months, reassured her their mother appeared fine to him.

Diane took a day off from work to assess the situation. Her stress level, always elevated as a result of a demanding job, shifted into high gear. When she arrived, her mother appeared to be her usual self, but when Diane took the time to look at the contents of her mother's refrigerator and noticed the stacks of unopened mail, she was forced to face the truth. A call to her brother left her frustrated; he felt she was overreacting. If she insisted on doing something, it was up to her—but it couldn't include having their mother come live with him, his wife and their four children. All this information was filtered by Diane's thalamus (a small gland in the brain that picks up sensory messages) and routed to the *amygdala* or appropriate parts of the *cortex.*

The amygdala is an area of the brain that processes emotional memories. It can activate just about every system in the body—not always accurately, but quickly. Smells and touch go directly to the amygdala, making a big impression and potentially triggering strong memories. The cortex gives data its meaning and tells the amygdala, "This is really something to panic about," or the prefrontal cortex can send an "all clear, calm down" message that the crisis is over.

In Diane's case, her brother's refusal to help reminded her of past experiences in which he had let her down, as well as experiences with her ex-husband who left when their only child died of leukemia. With her amygdala sounding alarms, other brain sites that act in more long-term ways went into action, including the *hippocampus*—the memory center that stores information and emotion. Diane could almost hear the increased hormonal response surging through her body as signals from the hypothalamus, pituitary and adrenal glands went into overdrive.

Epinephrine (adrenaline) from the adrenal glands made her heart pump faster and her lungs work harder. Her stress might not involve getting out of the way of a speeding car, but her adrenals weren't designed to think, only act. Their job is to flood her body with oxygen and insure that her senses are on hyperalert—the classic "stress" response. As hormones poured into her muscles, her digestive system, which is a nonessential system in an emergency, shut down. Diane found herself nauseous and struggling with a typical "lighten-the-load" response (vomit, urinate or defecate).

While all this was taking place, her adrenals simultaneously released extra cortisol and other glucocorticoids to make sure she would be able to convert enough sugar into energy. Nerve cells pumped out norepinephrine, tensing her muscles and sharpening her senses. Her body was prepared for major action, but for Diane there was no place to go.

Nevertheless, indecision about what to do, coupled with resistance from her mother at the suggestion of moving from her home, meant Diane's emergency "stress response" would continue. It kept her epinephrine and norepinephrine levels high—elevating risk to her arteries and increasing her already high family risk of heart disease.[7]

Further, her unresolved anxiety kept her glucocorticoids in circulation, weakening her immune system (she picked up a cold that was going around the office). Bone loss increased, her reproductive hormones were impacted, and her memory worsened. Adrenal hormones short-circuit the cells in the hippocampus, making it difficult to remember and/or organize thinking. When it hangs around too long, cortisol can kill millions of brain cells, including vital memory cells in the hippocampus. At work, Diane was chastised by her boss for overlooking an important memo.

Diane's instinct to pace the floor was good—exercise does help normalize out-of-control hormones. But her choice to drown her sorrows in high-octane caffeinated coffee and her increasingly shallow breaths made matters worse. Even though her adrenaline levels eventually dropped, the cortisol she released lasted much longer. Elevated levels of cortisol through the years have devastating effects on the body. It is the only hormone that increases in the body with age.

If Diane doesn't find a way to reduce her stress response, high cortisol levels will increase her blood sugar by up to 50 percent, weakening the immune system and increasing the chance for cancer and infectious diseases. It has already altered her sleep patterns. (She awakens at 2:30 A.M.) Abnormal levels are associated with chronic fatigue, fibromyalgia, depression, panic disorders and PMS. Protein synthesis, the activity of insulin, thyroid, dehydroepiandosterone (DHEA) and testosterone are all affected. Incidentally, Diane's concern over her weight and the stress she feels about what and how much she is eating is also increasing cortisol! Because she has modified her insulin production, fat will be increasingly deposited around her waist, indicating insulin resistance and consequent health risks.

Diane made an appointment with her doctor because of escalating menopause symptoms. Her hot flashes were keeping her up at night and embarrassing her at work. The unrelenting anxiety resulted in her first panic attack. She only vaguely mentioned her mother to her doctor. He wrote a prescription for hormone replacement therapy, reassuring her that she would not increase her breast cancer risk if she stayed on it for only three or four years; he failed to mention any cardiac risk. The prescription was for the lowest dose, but after a month it was doubled since her symptoms had not changed. He added a prescription of Zoloft because of its effectiveness with panic disorders.

Neither Diane nor her doctor considered another option—that years of stress culminating in this latest crisis may have resulted in maladaptive adrenal functioning. From a functional medicine viewpoint, this is a critical consideration. It is possible that Diane's adrenal glands are so overworked that they will be unable to respond effectively—a condition known as adrenal "burnout" or "adrenopause." Cortisol levels are intertwined with complaints of fatigue, arthritis and menstrual irregularities that look like "menopause." Imbalance of DHEA, also produced by the adrenals, and thus affected by chronic stress, has been associated with depression, insulin resistance, panic disorder and obesity, among other health issues.

Some natural support for times of high stress

Natural products that can be helpful for stress relief will be discussed thoroughly in future chapters. However, it seems appropriate to consider some basic choices here. Stress takes its toll, and it depletes vitamin resources, particularly the B-complex.

A "stress" B-complex will include vitamin C. Studies are investigating the possibility that an excess of 18 grams of inositol (an "unofficial" member of the B vitamins) might be a natural agent for panic attacks with none of the side effects.[8] Research measuring the effects of sustained stress on military combatants and others enduring severe circumstances demonstrated a measurable loss of magnesium and a rise in oxidative stress intensity, illustrating the need for antioxidant vitamins.[9] This and other research reveal the need for extra magnesium and inositol during particularly stressful times. The following Supplement Facts shows valuable information regarding B-complex vitamins.

Supplement Facts

Serving Size
Servings Per Container

	Amount Per Serving		% Daily Value
Vitamins and minerals with established Recommended Daily Intakes (RDI)	Range	Mg or IU	%
Thiamine (as thiamine mononitrate) **B$_1$** (see [A])	15–50	mg	%
Riboflavin **B$_2$** (see [B])	15–50	mg	%
Niacin (as a combination of niacinamide and not more than 10 mg niacin per day) **B$_3$** (see [C])	50–500	mg	%
Pantothenic acid (as D-calcium pantothenate) **B$_5$** (see [D])	100–500	mg	%
Vitamin **B$_6$** (as pyridoxine hydrochloride) (see [E])	20–100	mg	%
Folate (as **folic acid**, 5-methyl tetrahydrofolate [5MTHF] or 5-formyltetrahydrofolate [5FTHF]) **B$_9$** (see [F])	200–800	mcg	%
Vitamin **B$_{12}$** (as cyanocobalamin)	100–1000	mcg	%
Biotin **B$_7$** (see [G])	50–500	mcg	%
Choline (as choline bitartrate)	50–500	mg	%
Inositol	50–500	mg	%
Para-amino benzoic acid (PABA)	10–50	mg	%
Vitamin C (as ascorbic acid)	100–250	mg	%

** Daily Value not established.

[A] **B₁** aids nervous system, muscles, heart and digestion. Sources: brewer's yeast, whole grains, dried beans, salmon, sunflower seeds

[B] **B₂** aids energy, nervous system, eyes and skin. Sources: almonds, cheese, chicken

[C] **Niacin** provides energy; made by body from amino acid tryptophan. Sources: brewer's yeast, turkey, halibut, swordfish, tuna, peanuts, green vegetables and beans

[D] **B₅** aids normal growth, development and energy. Sources: all meats, whole grain, blue cheese, corn, eggs, lobster, nuts, mushrooms

[E] **B₆** helps metabolize amino acids; assists brain function, energy, stress, muscle tension, cramping/PMS. Sources: brewer's yeast, brown rice, cauliflower, walnuts, wheat germ, eggs, chicken, carrots

[F] **Folic acid** promotes normal red blood cells; aids Alzheimer's protection. Sources: barley, fruits, green leafy vegetables, added to flour and cereal

[G] **B₇** helps break down amino acids, carbohydrates and fats. Sources: almonds, peanuts, soybeans, bananas

WHEN STRESS MAKES YOU SICK

It is unfortunate that Diane had no social support system; having someone to talk to can be a wonderful, natural way to reduce the stress response. It is unlikely that her course of HRT and Zoloft will be very helpful. The risk/benefit profile of the HRT and even the Zoloft will not be in her favor. Unfortunately, it will probably take just enough of an edge off her misery that she will continue taking them. However, her altered adrenal function will remain a problem, escalating her cardiovascular risk, increasing her aches and pains and interrupting her sleep with all the consequences that result from such a scenario.

"Stress junkies"

There are other categories of people who are apt to find stress levels out of control. Some create a "crisis of the moment" to avoid reevaluation of their life situation or to escape having to face truths about themselves that are more easily suppressed. I've had a few clients in my therapy practice that created crisis and stress in order to feel *something* that would confirm they were alive—and coincidentally, let them receive sympathy and attention from others who wondered if there was a black cloud that followed this person around.

Others appear to *thrive* on their "adrenaline rush," unaware of the damage they are doing to their body. They could be called "stress junkies." The stress chemicals coursing through a "stress junkie's" body provide the punch needed to skip breakfast, work fourteen hours and then throw a dinner party for twelve of their closest friends. Taking on too much work, being a perfectionist or working with other "stress junkies" is guaranteed to set off the right alarm bells and prepare the body for gargantuan tasks. The days of using the "high" of stress as a mood-altering device are numbered, but addictive. The attempt to live this way for a sustained length of time frequently results in pent-up, unresolved anger and frustration, living right on the edge, which easily spills over. But the day of reckoning inevitably comes. For most, the bottom has fallen out the day they find they can't get out of bed, or they spend their coffee break hidden in the office broom closet, shedding uncontrollable tears.

Sometimes coming to terms with stress requires a good honest look at one's self, rather than a sole focus on the externals of your life. You may find that you feel emotionally powerless over some of your behavior; admonitions to "be calm" are likely to create more stress for the effort. It is OK to say, "This is a problem that I must have the courage to look at and take baby steps to change." Lyra and I—two self-identified "stress junkies"—give you permission to share the journey to peace with us.

COPING WITH STRESS

Undoing the damage of too much external or internal stress is not like getting over the flu. The process takes a while, and it involves some of the most benign of interventions. While the option exists to change jobs or trim a few things off your schedule by reprioritizing, most of us can count on stress continuing to be an impacting part of our lives. Like Diane, there will be brothers who expect you to take care of things, spouses who, at the very least, disappoint you, children who don't always do what they are supposed to, and the unrelenting pace of modern life. We can't eliminate stress, so we must learn to resist it where we can and learn to live with it in ways that don't hurt us.

We have already discussed important elements that contribute to stress release: therapeutic nutrition, exercise and the importance of social support. Their effects are overlapping. The stress response gives you energy to respond to a crisis. You can take that energy and literally work it off by walking or going to the gym—unless you are at the burnout stage, when less exercise is called for. A vital mechanism of exercise that reduces stress is the production and release of natural opiates known as endorphins.

And, as the UCLA study that follows confirms, people with an active and satisfying social network handle life's ups and down better, especially when they can laugh together. Organizing life so there is time for play and leisure activities is restorative.

Other simple interventions that work against stress include getting enough rest and relaxation, which go a long way in increasing your ability to handle whatever comes your way. Relaxation techniques, be they physical or mental, are valuable interventions that reduce the harmful effects of stress. Yoga has been mentioned previously. It is effective because of its ability to center and calm, as well as its encouragement to focus on breathing. Just breathing deeply can quell a racing heart and quiet you down. There are no side effects or financial costs for this very powerful intervention that can be done anywhere. Once you learn how, you will find it impossible to be anxious at the same time you are breathing deeply, slowly and regularly.

The restorative actions of prayer and meditation are also well researched. Meditation at a hormonal level counteracts the fight-or-flight response, slows the metabolism of red blood cells and suppresses the production of cytokines—proteins that generate pro-inflammatory responses in the body. The focus on breathing that is recommended during meditation keeps negative, distracting thoughts away. Massage and aromatherapy (with rose and lavender scents) are additional calming techniques that help relieve stress.

A gender difference

Women and men handle stress on the job differently. Women are more likely to get repetitive strain injuries, suffer from irritable bowel syndrome, headaches (especially in the thirty- to thirty-nine-year-old range), anxiety and depression. Men experience elevation in blood pressure. While women find their stress hormones rise at home and fall at work, men find work more stressful. I didn't need to tell you that, did I?

An interesting study from UCLA has demonstrated that women use friendships to lower their stress. In addition to the "fight-or-flight" stress response, women appear to have a number of responses to stressful events. The researchers theorized that the hormone oxytocin, which is enhanced by estrogen in women and reduced by testosterone in men, encourages women to tend to children and gather with other women when stressed.[10]

This response, called "tending and befriending," stimulates increased release of oxytocin, which produces a calming effect. The authors maintain this unique feminine response has been overlooked because 90 percent of all studies on stress have been done on men. They speculate that a woman's social ties may be a factor in reducing risk to disease, and it helps explain why women tend to live longer than men. One study found that over a nine-year period, women who had the most friends cut their risk of early death by more than 60 percent. A review of the Harvard Medical School Nurses' Health Study confirmed that women who had the most friends as they aged had fewer physical impairments and thus more reason to live a joyful life. This proved true even after the death of a spouse.[11]

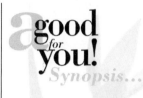

1. Do you exercise excessively or not at all? What have you told yourself about this?

2. What kind of activities did you enjoy as a kid? Are there aspects you can reproduce in your present life?

3. What one thing can you do to increase your physical activity and relieve stress? Will you do it? Why or why not?

4. Do you feel worse after exercise? Consider the possibility of adrenal burnout as the cause.

5. Are you a stress junkie? How would your life be different if you weren't?

6. What did your family have to say about people who run on adrenaline? Did it make them seem important? Crazy?

7. Can you identify the people, places, things, commitments or responsibilities in your life that cause you continuous worry, fret and stress? Make a list. Can you entertain the possibility that these involvements can be managed in a way that is less draining?

PART III
The Action

You can't sleep; hot flashes are driving you back to the hormone replacement therapy you stopped three months ago. You aren't a crusader; you just want to feel good. There is only so much you are willing to do. "Just give it to me fast and simple," you say.

We intend to do just that, but we need to go one step further. A list of safe, natural products is easy to provide, but how do you know which one to buy?

Chapter twelve takes you on a virtual tour of a health food store. Through a process of elimination, you can be certain that what you buy will not only be what it says it is, but also the correct product for you.

Once you know what to look for, chapter thirteen will supply the minimum you should consider for both menopause and healthy aging.

Should symptoms require a more specific approach, chapter fourteen will give suggestions for natural relief.

Since midlife misery is often attributable to something other than menopause, chapter fifteen suggests what else might be causing you to be tired, not sleeping or otherwise unwell.

12

an informed trip to the health food store

Wе have asked you to exercise your left brain (logical reasoning) in making sense of the complicated impact on your body of metabolites of estrogen. This chapter asks for a billboard of lights, camera and action as you make connection with your creative, right-brain imaginative parts. We are going to take you on a virtual tour of a health food store. You will, of course, retain access to your left brain, because by now you have become a *critical thinker* and will be calling upon it to analyze and sort information.

In chapter thirteen you will study and scrutinize interventions available to relieve discomfort triggered by menopause and/or just getting older. You will develop a list of products/foods you decide might help you, based on your unique pattern of symptoms. But you have lots of questions. How do you find the most effective formula to meet your personal need? Is one brand better than another? Where do you go to purchase them? We wanted to answer the questions before you asked them so that you will not be frustrated in your action steps that follow.

A VIRTUAL TOUR

The *brrrrrring* of the alarm signals it is time to get up. You don't mind, because quality sleep has been elusive. You have tossed and turned throughout the night, throwing off the covers, opening the window and listening to the frogs that croak from some mysterious spot in your yard. *Good for You!* lies beside your bed, filled with underlines, *yes* and *get this* scribbled in the margin. A corner is turned down marking your place. Tucked in the back is the envelope that once contained your health insurance bill; it seemed an appropriate (or maybe just handy) notepad to jot down the products you have decided to purchase.

Your bleary eyes pick out your "uniform" for natural food shopping. It is a uniform in the sense that, if memory serves you correctly, the last time you tried to purchase a natural product, you were defeated by the sheer numbers, the outrageous promises and the bubblegum-chewing clerk who practically followed you to your car insisting she had everything you needed for *what ails you*. Today you will be prepared; you are armed for action. You top off an outfit of stretch pants (for easy bending) and your best walking shoes (for spending hours on your feet) with your travel vest—the one with fifty visible pockets and ten hidden ones. The final touch, just in case, is a waist pack, big enough to hold a nutritional bar should the going get really tough, a bottle of water, your reading glasses, your kid's magnifying glass from his bug-looking set and, of course, your dog-eared copy of *Good for You!*

You have carefully stashed your cheat sheets in the various pockets. Your list for the criteria to which a company needs to adhere in order to ensure safety of its products is in the lower left pocket. An FDA update on natural products and a chart containing herb/drug interactions is tucked into the upper left one. Questions to ask the store manager regarding manufacturers and a notepad to take down numbers of distributors or manufacturers, should you need more information, is easily reached in the right pocket. And finally, the personal list of products that you have determined are right for you from chapter thirteen is safely zippered into the hidden inner pouch. You are ready to be an informed consumer!

You arrive at the natural foods market, a drug store or specialty supplement store and take a moment to assess the lay of the land. The terror of the job is brought home once again as you see people drifting in and out of the aisles, their eyes much like deer who have become mesmerized by oncoming headlights. Aisle after aisle of vitamins, minerals, protein powders, digestive enzymes, amino acids and herbs in capsules, powders, liquids, pellets and packets are enough to make you sick in your pursuit of health. For a moment you panic.

Maybe you should have gone on the Internet again or succumbed to your neighbor's multilevel marketing company. But then you remember trying to sort through all those claims. How do you know what to believe, or can you? You fortify yourself with a bite of your nutrition bar, take a swig of water and march onward—you are up to the task because you know from *Good for You!* what to look for and what to ask!

Making the buying of natural products doable

Accomplishing your goal of purchasing a safe and reasonably effective product or formula requires:

1. A definition of *safe* and *effective*
2. An understanding of the criteria that determine safety and efficacy
3. A way of identifying if a product meets the criteria
4. A user-friendly checklist for selecting a product

Just what is a safe, effective natural product supposed to do? It is obviously different from a pharmacological drug prescribed by your physician, which kills a specific bacteria or is prescribed for a very precise job. Natural medicines frequently have a broader goal and are capable of restoring balance and improving function (mental, emotional, physical, sexual) with the hope of promoting optimal performance, longevity and wellness, as well as favorably impacting disease risk. They can also supplement deficits in the diet.

Natural medicines are not *silver bullets* or "pills for ills." Outrageous claims and promises feed fear and build false hopes. In fact, this truth gives you your first criterion for making a selection: Eliminate any product that promises it is the breakthrough answer or miracle for an illness or health issue.

something *to think about*

Eliminate any product that promises it is the breakthrough answer or miracle for an illness or health issue.

You must be realistic regarding your expectations, especially if your preference is "to only do this much," as we will discuss in the next two chapters. Natural-based therapies are *preferred* because they are developed to restore health and improve function. For example, vitamins and minerals make up for deficits from a mishandled food supply, poor eating pattern or a metabolic imbalance that results in nutrients being in short supply.

WHAT IS A DIETARY SUPPLEMENT?

In 1994, the Dietary Supplement Health and Education Act (DSHEA) defined dietary supplements as foods.[1] Such products are intended to supplement the diet or increase total dietary intake and contain one or more of the following: vitamins, minerals, amino acids, herbs or other botanicals that can be concentrates, metabolites, constituents, extracts or some combination of these. Not included in this definition but commonly found in supplements are animal-derived products and hormones. Within these categories, products may be pure single entities of known or unknown chemical components or mixtures in which all or none of the components may be known or unknown. The possible combinations boggle the mind. Consider the examples of dietary supplements in the following chart:

examples of dietary supplements

DIETARY SUPPLEMENT	EXAMPLES
Vitamins	B-complex (there are 12), such as vitamins B_1, B_2, niacin or folic acid (water soluble); vitamins A, D, E and K (fat soluble)
Minerals	Calcium, magnesium, sodium, potassium, selenium, chromium, vanadium, copper, zinc
Amino acids	Lysine, tyrosine, N-acetylcysteine (NAC), tryptophan
Herbs	Peppermint, chamomile, St. John's wort, kava, echinacea, goldenseal, ginseng, valerian, black cohosh, chasteberry (a.k.a. Vitex), licorice, lavender
Enzymes	Pancreatic enzymes from animals or fruit like pineapple and papaya (containing substances like protease, lipase, amylase, etc.)
Animal-tissue-derived substances	Liver, adrenal and thymus tissue from beef, pig and sheep glands and organs
Nature-identical hormones and analogues	Progesterone cream synthesized from yams, estrogen concentrated from soy, Dehydroepiandrosterone (DHEA) concentrated from yam
Natural metabolites	Antioxidants like CoQ_{10}; phytonutrients like flavonoids from citrus or pomegranate (ellagic acid); carotenoids (alpha and beta carotenes); polycosinols from sugar cane
Mixtures	Products containing two or more ingredients from the same or assorted categories of dietary supplements: multivitamin mineral with or without an herbal base; traditional herbal formulations from India (Ayurvedic), China or Native North America; novel mixtures of herbs, vitamins and enzymes.

Natural product chemists identify the molecules within foods and herbs that demonstrate potential to make a difference in how you feel and/or to change physiology and chemistry in your body, like cholesterol or hormone levels. Supplements can selectively reinforce parts of the body that need more of a particular substance that might be difficult to get from the small amounts in food alone. When concentrated, they can enhance what is present in food or complement the diet by enhancing a food's potential to intentionally influence physical function.

For example, B vitamins are highly recommended for their ability to support liver function and combat stress. Most multivitamins include a combination of B vitamins that are present in up to a thousand times the amount they occur in food. Does that sound scary? Don't worry, they are water soluble and do not accumulate in the body. As is true of most supplements, the benefits when given as a group or individually are tied to how much you take.

The B vitamin niacin occurs in the diet in micrograms (1,000 micrograms equals 1 milligram). If your health practitioner recommends you take it (and periodically checks your liver function) to improve your cholesterol balance, he or she may recommend doses of 1,000 mg to 3,000 mg per day. Since high doses can cause itching and hot flushes, it is sometimes prescribed in sustained-release doses. You simply could not eat enough food containing niacin to reach the levels needed to affect cholesterol positively.

Cod liver oil is another good example of the benefits of supplementation. It is a great source of vitamins A and D as well as "healthy fats" known as omega-3 fatty acids (EPA/DHA). However, if you were to try and supplement with cod liver oil as your primary source of EPA/DHA, you risk consuming dangerous levels of vitamins A and D. Neither of these are water soluble; therefore, they can accumulate in the liver.

The dosage of vitamin D and directions for use are regulated by the FDA. This serves as a reminder that it is just as important to follow directions with supplements as you do with prescription drugs. On the other hand, if you decide to have fish be your source of omega-3, you may risk ingesting excess mercury, a known environmental contaminant. A study in the *New England Journal of Medicine* reported a direct association between the risk of heart attacks and mercury levels.[2] If you are uncertain about the origin of your fish, a better choice may be to take EPA/DHA in capsules that come with proof they are mercury free. This will also eliminate the worry of consuming excess vitamins A and D.

something ^to^*think about*

Eliminate spontaneous purchases that you have not investigated for safety and benefits and that do not address a specific problem you have identified as a personal concern.

So what does this mean to you? It should present a caution to you to not add to the possibility of harm by deciding to "browse" through a health food store and buy what looks interesting. When you search for products, search by informed *need*. Eliminate spontaneous purchases that you have not investigated for safety and benefits and that do not address a specific problem you have identified as a personal concern.

WHAT ARE THE CRITERIA FOR SAFETY AND EFFICACY?

The intention of a drug is to treat a health condition or relieve specific symptoms. The intention of a food is to nourish and support the body or improve its function, generally or specifically. The safety of both is tied to how much you can consume without side effects or risk of an adverse event. A special danger lies in combining dietary supplement products with over-the-counter (OTC) or prescription medications. Ingredient safety is also directly associated with freedom from environmental pollutants, whether they come from the air, water, earth, unfriendly bacteria or the manufacturing process.

How effective a product is—its efficacy—depends on preparation and dosage. Supplement companies are limited by law in what they can tell you about the actual health benefits of most natural products because that would make them sound like a drug—and they are licensed as a food product. A company is limited to structure and function statements with the recommended dose.

For example, omega-3 fatty acids, EPA/DHA, can act like a natural "anti-inflammatory" agent—in essence, a painkiller. This, however, would be an illegal statement for a manufacturer to include. They can say EPA/DHA supports healthy eicosanoid production (function) and cell membrane fluidity (structure). If you are not familiar with the significance of these biochemical pathways and "functions," let me explain that it translates as *pain relief.*

The vast majority of natural products are safe to consume when you know that the manufacturer performs due diligence and complies with FDA food regulations and there is good scientific evidence that the ingredient has human value. The real consumer concerns revolve around beneficial dose. Safety and efficacy can only be thoroughly understood when you take the time to gather the science. A reputable company will comply with DSHEA, offering a thoroughly tested product to insure safety and accurate "structure and function" information. It will also find a way to give you the references from the scientific literature, which will help you sort through additional concerns you might have such as the unique "beneficial dose" for you within the bounds of safety.

Safety regulations

All dietary supplement manufacturers by law must adhere to *good manufacturing practice* (GMP) specifications just as rigorous as those affecting any food preparation manufacturer. The goal of the dietary supplement GMP regulations is to insure that what is on the label is in the product every time a batch is manufactured, that there is no contamination and that it disintegrates (to be appropriately absorbed) in thirty minutes after consumption.

In short, it is not a valid criticism to say that the supplement industry is "unregulated." It is regulated. However, it is the choice of the company whether they wish to go further and adopt standards required for over-the-counter drugs or for pharmaceutical manufacturing. While there is no obligation for them to do so, there are dietary supplement companies and manufacturers who, in the spirit of excellence and concern over inferior and possibly injurious products, also voluntarily choose to do just that.

There are ongoing efforts from consumers and the government to increase regulations within the industry. (See Appendix B.) Since the DSHEA regulations stipulate that dietary supplements are food, the burden of proof for safety rests with the FDA after the supplement is in the marketplace. The FDA can only intervene if a consumer complains. This does not mean you are at the mercy solely of a company's word or lack thereof. A good company will have assays backed by internal and independent laboratories that confirm what they put on their label. The store, supplier or company should have no problem obtaining such proof for you.

Companies that make good products make a very big deal about what they do to insure purity of ingredients, efficient absorption and positive outcome. If you are getting the message that safety of supplements depends on the integrity of both company and manufacturer, you are absolutely correct. Ask how long the company has been in business. What do retailers say about it? Do health practitioners hold it in high regard and recommend it? In combination with the availability of assays to confirm label claims, positive recommendations suggest that within the company there are good formulators who design the products and experts in the field (versus the laboratory only) who participate in product

something *to think about*

Eliminate any product not made by a manufacturer with a reputation you can trust.

safety and development. Eliminate any product not made by a manufacturer with a reputation you can trust.

CRITERIA FOR BOTANICAL SAFETY AND QUALITY

Of all the dietary supplements, there are more opportunities for contamination, mislabeling and false claims with herbs, also called *botanicals*, than with any other class of natural agents. The problem lies in the fact that methods for testing the presence of specific herbs and their active ingredients in finished products are still being developed. The science has yet to catch up with the tradition. With many other classes of dietary supplements, assays are reliable, and acceptable ranges of ingredients are well known. Vitamins and minerals with established Recommended Daily Intakes (RDI), for instance, will have that information included in their labels.

Besides good manufacturing practices (GMP), a responsible company will add another level of surveillance when working with herbs, sometimes referred to as *good plant practice* (GPP). GPP requires rigorous plant screening using several methods to establish the plant's identity. A spelled-out process of quality assurance and control (QA/QC) supplies absolute proof of the genus, species and plant part. Latin is used because the names are constant, whereas common names vary. Appropriate labeling includes common and Latin names of each herb.

something
to think about

Eliminate botanical products that do not clearly list the Latin genus, species name and plant part in their labeling.

One genus can have many species. For example, black cohosh is the most commonly used plant for perimenopausal symptoms. The genus and species that appears to result in the greatest improvement is black cohosh, *Cimicifuga racemosa*, recently renamed *Actaea racemosa*. The benefit is mainly derived from the roots and rhizomes. There are at least four species grown in the United States, with other species grown in China and other parts of the world. The only way you can determine whether or not the black cohosh you buy is one that is likely to be most helpful is to find the Latin genus, species name and plant part(s) listed on the label.

Common name listings such as black cohosh root, peppermint leaf, garlic, Chin pi (a Chinese name) and Ashwagandha (Ayurvedic name) are inadequate. A company that uses common names only and/or that doesn't list the plant part or uses foreign names is one you should avoid.

POWDERS, CRUDE AND STANDARDIZED EXTRACTS

In general, unprocessed herbal powders are the least potent and the most likely to be contaminated with pesticides and toxic metals. Unprocessed plants are those that are cultivated or gathered from the fields or the wild and then dried, powdered and, hopefully, treated to eliminate microbial growth or pests. To the uninformed, a list of several herbal powders in a product may appear impressive. However, the amount of powder that a person would need to consume to gain benefit can be enormous compared to what is in a capsule or pill. Rarely, with few exceptions, are there enough active ingredients present to produce a clinically effective response. Since herbal powders are inexpensive, companies can easily afford to include them, giving the product the allure of herbs without the punch.

Ginkgo leaf (*ginkgo biloba*) is a great example of an herb that should not be taken as a powder, but is frequently sold as such to reduce cost. Gingko has circulatory and memory benefits, and many women find it helpful for menopausal mental "fogginess" if the correct preparation is used. The part that does the work is found in the leaves in tiny amounts. The active ingredients, *ginkoflavonglycosides* and *terpene lactones,* are obtained by concentrating them from large amounts of ginkgo leaves. Thirty to forty pounds of leaves are required to yield one pound of a clinically active preparation capable of supplying a beneficial dose of these important phytochemicals. The finished material is known as a standardized extract. It is "standardized" because it contains the levels of ginkoflavonglycosides and terpene lactones known to be present in amounts associated with the benefits of gingko based on human clinical trials.

There is no getting around the fact that when dealing with herbal products you must be knowledgeable about the best preparation and beneficial dose for your specific health issue. Here you must depend on someone who is trained or experienced or exercise your left brain and do some reading. Do not panic. We will give you your best options for the hormonal and aging issues you are most likely dealing with in the next two chapters.

Consider *this...* Dietary supplements are used most frequently by older individuals and those who report having more healthful lifestyles.[3]

SELECTING A PRODUCT THAT IS SAFE AND THAT WORKS

Ultimately what you want to know is if the product is safe and will work. The truth is every ingredient in every product you pick up or read about comes with some science to justify its presence in the marketplace. In that sense, all those bottles and potions have some validity for being there. They have behind them a legitimate purpose—it is just that some are more legitimate than others. And that leads us to our next criterion of selection: Eliminate products with ingredients whose science or traditional use is weak.

something
to think about

Eliminate products with ingredients whose science or traditional use is weak.

You will find as you become more familiar with natural medicine that some ingredients have more human research than others; some have only been demonstrated to work in media-cultures in a laboratory or with animals. There are products that are formulated because they have been used effectively for generations, while others are new inventions or purified extracts from foods or plants with minimal human research, but they show promise. Manufacturers, distributors and those who sell products must provide actual research that discusses its history and science. Every ingredient has a story, and you must become an investigative reporter to uncover what it is.

WHAT DOES THE LABEL TELL YOU?

At this point, my suggestion is that you take a moment to grab one of your vitamin or botanical bottles and follow along. The DSHEA act not only defined what a dietary supplement is, but it also spelled out label requirements. Currently a company does not have to include cautionary warnings or suggestions for proper use. Even the quantity of each ingredient is not necessary. What is required is the descriptive name of the product stating that it is a supplement, the name and place of business of the distributor, packer or manufacturer, a complete list of ingredients and net contents of the product.[4]

What follows is an example of a label that a natural supplement manufacturer might produce. It exceeds the minimal standards and serves as a positive example of what you should be looking for. The label is your clue as to the integrity of the company. It and the technical information it contains are the beginning of establishing product credibility and quality. You should consider it a strong and telling message. Take a look at your sample and see how it compares. Our example is a black cohosh product we will simply call *Black Cohosh and More.* (Note: The name is fictitious although the information is exactly as printed.) The label is divided into three segments as follows:

a three-panel label

STRUCTURE FUNCTION CLAIMS	NAME OF PRODUCT	SUPPLEMENT FACTS BOX
	Black Cohosh and More Motherwort and lemon balm extracts Vegetarian Herbal Supplement (see [A]) 60 tablets (see [B])	

[A] Required to be listed as a supplement
[B] Not required, but helpful in cost consideration

The following is a representation of a good Structure Function Claim box, the left panel of the label. It contains information not always required by law, but necessary for your proper evaluation of a natural supplement.

structure function claim box

Black Cohosh and More supports the menopausal woman with a unique botanical blend that features premium black cohosh extract, an herb traditionally used to maintain healthy female hormone balance. Black cohosh is combined with motherwort and lemon balm, herbs traditionally used to ease tension and support relaxation (see [C]). **These statements have not been evaluated by the Food and Drug Administration. This product is not intended to diagnose, treat, cure or treat any disease (see [D]).**

Directions: Take one tablet twice daily or as directed by your healthcare practitioner. Warning: Do not use if pregnant or nursing (see [E]).

Caution: Keep out of the reach of children (see [F]).

Storage: Keep tightly closed in a cool, dry place (see [G]).

Does Not Contain: Wheat, gluten, corn protein, yeast, soy, animal or dairy products or artificial colors, sweeteners or preservatives.

[C] Not required but detail about traditional use and the rationale for inclusion are given (structure/function). No misleading claims or generalizations that all ingredients do what the most active one does.
[D] Required
[E] Not required, but clearly stated instructions for proper use
[F] Not required, but clearly important for safe use.
[G] Not required, but clearly important for safe use.

The following is a representation of a good Supplement Facts box, the right panel of the label. It contains the recommended daily intakes (RDI) of herbs with their genus/species and preparation. Nonessential ingredients like herbs, enzymes, antioxidants, metabolites and isolated substances for which a specific individual amount is listed are included under "other ingredients."

Supplement Facts

Serving Size   1 tablet
Servings Per Container   60

	Amount Per Serving	% Daily Value
Only RDI nutrients (minerals, vitamins) are listed in this area. This area may not appear if vitamins and minerals are absent from the formula.		
Black cohosh rhizome extract (*Actaearacemosa syn Cimicifuga racemosa*) standardized to contain 2.5% (2 mg) triterpene glycosides as 27-deoyactein (see [A])	80 mg	**
Motherwort Aerial Parts 6:5:1 Extract (*Leomurus cardiaca*) (see [B])	100 mg	**
Lemon Balm Leaf 5:1 Extract (*Melissa officianalis*) (see [B])	50 mg	**

**Daily Value not established

Other ingredients (for example, natural excipients): Dicalcium phosphate, starch, stearic acid, silica, magnesium stearate and modified cellulose coating

Distributed by XXXXXXXXXX
Makers of Professional Quality Supplements
Xxxxx, California (see [C])
Lot # (see [D])   Product # (see [D])

[A] Required: a complete list of ingredients and net contents of the product. A precise description of ingredients: common name, plant part, genus and species. (If this were a vitamin/mineral product the recommended daily intake RDI would be included.)

[B] Common name and Latin genus/species. Latin name insures safety.

[C] Required: name and place of manufacturer

[D] Not required: lot and product number. However, important to insure safety.

The label for our Black Cohosh and More goes far beyond what is asked of a nutritional supplement company—no extraordinary claims are made, appropriate warnings and cautions are included, and a means of tracing the batch is available. Thus, a quick but careful perusal of a label gives you another reason for eliminating or selecting the product. Eliminate any product whose label is more hype than business and doesn't contain more information than what is currently required.

something
to think about

Eliminate any product whose label is more hype than business.

Did all three of the label panels on your product exceed DSHEA standards? Are you clear about the information a good label should include? Are you feeling more confident that you can make a good choice? Do you still have some doubts about using herbal products? If you do, read Appendix B. It contains additional information about safety and oversight of dietary supplements and suggests some additional reading sources for you.

Evaluating your decision

By using our elimination criteria and studying the label, our virtual shopper located products she feels confident will be safe and effective. In fact, she selected several products that meet her standards, and now she must pick between seemingly equal choices. It may be that, all things being equal, there is nothing else to do but choose one because she likes the color of the label! She may, however, decide to look a little deeper.

Our virtual shopper could request additional written literature that elaborates on the company and their more extensive rationale for inclusion of each ingredient. She could ask about the exclusive procedures the company uses for establishing species authenticity and purity. It may be important for her to know if they have a policy that excludes endangered plant species and supports a sustainable harvest.

What if she makes her selection but finds it doesn't do what she wanted or needed it to do? First, she must realize that, unlike an aspirin that works quickly, many botanicals require a period of time before efficacy can be determined. They are influencing body function, and that does not happen in an instant.

Let's say that she is realistic about giving her black cohosh product time to work, and it doesn't. Does that mean that black cohosh (or any herbal product) is ineffective, and she should give up and go back to HRT? No, what it means is that because of individualization, the particular formulation purchased may not work for her. If such a thing happens to you, you can become your own *health sleuth*. It is all right to experiment to find out what happens if you take the product on a full stomach. What happens on an empty one? At night? In the morning? If you exercise a little more or add a cup of soy milk every day? Could another company's product prove more effective?

What the future holds

Government officials and others claim to be concerned over safety of dietary supplements centering around "continually evolving patterns of dietary supplement use and potential interactions with other consumed substances." While the concern *sounds* important, a more accurate rendering is not safety as much as the fact that dietary supplements have become big business. Total sales are estimated at $15.7 billion per year.[5] The FDA estimates that more than twenty-nine thousand different dietary supplements are now available with one thousand new ones added annually.[6]

In Europe most natural products are manufactured in a separate but parallel track alongside conventional pharmaceuticals, and the market is three times larger than in the United States. There is little chance that "plant" medicines will be brought to market as "drugs" in this country, considering the estimated $231 million required to do so and the fact that they can't be patented. This has led to accusations that drug research has focused on patented "synthetic" versions of medications and avoided production and research of natural alternatives.

HERB/SUPPLEMENT AND DRUG INTERACTIONS

While there are legitimate safety concerns for the fast-growing alternative medicine industry, it is important to keep the danger in perspective. It is true there have been unscrupulous or merely careless manufacturers with tragic results involving herbal medicines. Such incidents do not come close to the risk of pharmaceutically prescribed drugs. A telling 1998 study reported, from databases reviewed from 1966 to 1996, that in 1994 alone there were 2,216,000 serious adverse drug reactions in hospitalized patients and 106,000 *fatal* drug adverse events. Adverse prescription drugs ranged between the fourth and sixth leading causes of death. Note that these events occurred under the direction of professionals in a hospital setting.[7] Leading painkillers (ibuprofen, Advil and Motrin) cause perforated ulcers that result in almost seventy thousand hospitalizations a year and sixteen thousand deaths. Bleeding occurs with no forewarning symptoms in 85 percent of cases.[8]

By comparison, problems with herbs or interactions of herbs and drugs, specifically, are rather low. Most of the time, an adverse herb reaction takes the form of a rash, gastrointestinal upset or headache. Discontinuing the herb resolves the problem. The most serious problems have been those that have resulted in liver damage, but this has been rare. In fact, generally the problem has not been with the herb but more a combination of a patient's present health condition and the drugs and herbs he or she is taking.

A review of the literature of possible interactions with the seven top-selling herbal medicines and prescribed drugs generated what was called a "sparse" result.[9]

herbal safety

THE SEVEN TOP-SELLING HERBS	COMMON USE	CAUTIONS AND SAFETY RECORD
Echinacea	Builds immunity	None
Saw palmetto	Prostate health	None
Kava	Anxiety and insomnia	Liver toxicity with a history of liver or alcohol problems; not to be taken by Parkinson patients taking levodopa or alprazolam
St. John's wort	Mild to moderate depression	Incompatible with antivirals by interfering with liver pathways; lowers blood concentrations of cyclosporin, amitriptyline, digoxin, indinavir, warfarin, phenprocoumon and theophylline; intermenstrual bleeding with oral contraceptives; not to be used with selective serotonin reuptake inhibitors
Ginkgo	Memory	Not to be used with warfarin; raises blood pressure when combined with a thiazide diuretic and should never be used with trazodone
Ginseng	Energy, immune function	Not be taken with warfarin
Garlic	Heart health	Not be taken with warfarin

While ephedra extract was not mentioned, it has been used by many women for weight loss and increased energy. Its use is highly discouraged because it can cause rapid heartbeat (tachycardia) and increased cardiovascular risk, which has resulted in stern warnings from the government against its use in weight loss products.[10] Ephedra is a classic example of a plant taken out of traditional context, in which it was not a problem—that is, in combination with other herbs, for short periods of time to open airways in cases of asthma, sinus and chest congestion for which it had positive effects.

All botanical and supplemental products have a physiological action. If they didn't, there would be no point in taking them. Herbal products can alter normal body functions (and abnormal ones); therefore, it is important to understand and become informed consumers, sensitive to the possibility of herb/food/supplement and drug interactions, just as we should be with the potentially more life-threatening interactions between prescription drugs.

Concerns about possible interactions of herbs and drugs are especially warranted when an herb or combination of herbs has a focused effect similar to the intended drug. A synergy and antagonism between herb(s) and drug(s) may produce additive effects, amplifying the effect of the drug. For example, it could inhibit drug absorption, increase elimination, alter drug metabolism or excretion time, cause drug retention or slow detoxification.

Protecting yourself

To protect yourself from adverse effects, follow these guidelines:

- Make sure you are honest about all the alternative approaches you are using by informing your prescribing physician and/or pharmacist.

- Take herbs and prescriptions at different times of the day.

- Be aware of plant allergies you have.

- Start with a low to moderate herb dose and work up.

Media attention, good and bad, will become an increasingly significant factor in generating consumer and clinician interest and will increase safety claims. Increasingly, scientific studies and clinical trials are becoming available (in English) to support efficacy and safety. Undoubtedly, the use of standardized extracts as a guarantee of quality and reliability will become a key element in brand building and reliance. Manufacturers in the United States are producing herbal products that have never been in existence before and for which there is no traditional use. The increased potency means you must be vigilant and aware of their use because of side effects in general and interactions with conventional medicines. This trend of combining several standardized extract ingredients is a uniquely contemporary phenomenon.

The following user-friendly checklist will be helpful to you when you decide to take your uniform for a shopping spree of healthful products. We recommend that you photocopy it and carry it with you to help you become an informed consumer.

YOUR USER-FRIENDLY CHECKLIST

Before you walk into a store

1. *Be prepared*
   What is your health goal?
   What ingredients are most apt to help?

When you walk into a store

2. *Eliminate products*
   Unrealistic promises or hype
   Fly-by-night manufacturer or poor reputation
   Ingredients without sound science or tradition
   Poor/minimal labeling

3. *Select products*
   Made for your age, sex and state of health
   With tradition and/or science to support your health goal
   With price points reflective of the benefit and quality expected

4. *Take note*
   Potential side effects?
   Potential for herb/supplement and drug interactions?
   Directions?

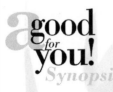
a **good** *for* **you!** *Synopsis…*

1. How does it feel to become a *Good for You!* safety sleuth?
2. Do you feel less intimidated? You should. You now have the tools for spotting questionable products through the process of elimination highlighted throughout the chapter. And you have your checklist!

13

i will only do this much: foundation supplements

We have noted how individual our responses to food, medicine and even exercise happen to be—physiologically we are all unique. We seem to have no problem accepting that what works metabolically for one person may not be helpful and may even be harmful for another. However, it appears more problematic to accept our psychological individuality. As you have surmised, Lyra and I are very different people. Yes, we are both Type A, disciplined and academically inclined. But if we are laying our cards out on the table, I am much less concerned about the need to occasionally pop an aspirin than Lyra is.

Lyra's world is health and natural health products and insuring that not only her body but also those with whom she comes in contact get what they need to function properly. My world is health and writing and trying as often as possible to land on the good side of what needs to be done—but I remain symbolically ready to "grab the aspirin" when pain or fatigue reach a certain point.

I would like to be more like Lyra. I am sure my body would love it, but the occasional slice of bacon, the freshness of Sonoma County bread and the longing for a night without hot flashes leave me vulnerable. Give me a "silver bullet" that you can prove will not do more harm than good, and I will consider it. Granted, I have had a lot more health issues to deal with than Lyra, and living with an allopathic physician—an obstetrician/gynecologist, no less—has not left me completely adverse to the promised quick fixes.

Those of you who are paying attention are probably saying to yourself, "Yeah, look where it got you—you're a litany of health issues." On bad days

I would agree; often what I deal with is made worse by my penchant for overwork and my failure to take care of my stress appropriately. On good days, I know that bugs, viruses, pesticides and the genes I carry leave some things out of my control. And there is no way to know what might have happened had I been exposed to good health alternatives earlier. In the meantime, illness happens.

DO WHAT YOU ARE WILLING TO DO

My point is, you have both Lyra's and my permission to admit that there is only so much you are willing to do. It is important that you know there are options, even if you decide not to select them for the time being. I must warn you that a wonderful thing about health is that little successes tend to motivate you on to bigger ones. So do what you can. We do not intend to let you off the hook completely, however. "I will only do this much" preferably involves some baby-step lifestyle changes and several different kinds of supplements.

something to think about

A wonderful thing about health is that little successes tend to motivate you on to bigger ones.

The intention of the next two chapters is to offer you real strategies and natural agents that have the potential to help you age well with lots of energy and calm your hot flashes, sweats, moodiness, aches and pains so you can function at a higher level. This is accomplished by supporting several organ and gland systems that directly and indirectly contribute to balanced hormone metabolism (good-girl/bad-girl estrogens).

Ultimately, a diet rich in a variety of fruits and vegetables, while limiting intake of animal protein and saturated fat, exercising until you sweat, honing coping skills and committing to a fully expressed life are the keys to healthy aging and an uneventful menopause. Indeed, this is a mouthful, a "life-full"—and it is an unachievable goal. Transformation comes about by enrolling in the process of self-examination and taking those baby steps. While you may never completely "arrive," you can get on the road. You may not be ready today, but this afternoon, you might reconsider. How about tomorrow? So, with this said, there are safe and effective interventions that hold the promise of helping you feel better quickly without mandating that you change every one of your eating and lifestyle habits.

THE WHOLE PERSON GOES THROUGH MENOPAUSE

At the moment you experience your first hot flash or mood swing, or when the doctor tells you that your bones are melting, the sum of who you are is going through menopause. This is why there is no such thing as a menopause silver bullet. Your whole body, mind and spirit are involved in "the change"—one pill is not going to "fix" it. The intensity, frequency and duration of symptoms are moderated by the health status of your entire body with a seasoning of genes thrown in for good measure.

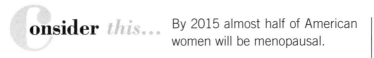

onsider *this...* By 2015 almost half of American women will be menopausal.

Menopause is neither a diseased nor a stable state. The changes at midlife that usher you into your "third age" involve multiple organ and gland systems. While it is a completely natural process, unless surgically induced or structural (your ovaries never developed), your body is in a dynamic state of hormonal flux every day, every hour. This hormonal roller-coaster ride affects mood and behavior, temperature control, your skin, memory and ability to sleep. Hormones are seriously influenced by the liver, adrenals, thyroid and the ability to maintain balanced blood sugar levels. This entire array of hormonal events and organ and glandular functions is influenced by select vitamins, minerals, botanicals, nonessential micronutrients and such.

Midlife and beyond fundamentals

To maximize the effectiveness of other natural interventions as well as provide symptom relief directly, you must begin by fortifying your diet with ample vitamins, minerals, essential fatty acids and select phytonutrients/phytochemicals concentrated from vegetables, fruits and legumes. Remember, foods that supply these vital nutrients are infrequently eaten even by the most health-conscious women. Fortification or enrichment should take the form of:

1. A high-quality multivitamin/mineral supplement
2. An emphasis on fish oils
3. A class of plant extracts known as phytoestrogens, or more correctly, phytochemicals that mimic or modify your hormones

Since phytoestrogens act like selective estrogen receptor modifiers (SERMs), henceforth we will call them phytoSERMs. Your foundation program is a "spill-over" intervention, meaning that it provides both direct symptom relief and protection against diseases of aging.

If you do nothing else, at least take a good quality multivitamin. Purchase a well-balanced formula that looks somewhat like the following:

identifying vitamin/mineral supplements you can trust

VITAMINS AND MINERALS WITH ESTABLISHED RECOMMENDED DAILY INTAKES (RDI)	AMOUNT PER SERVING RANGE MG/IU	WHAT YOU SHOULD KNOW
FAT SOLUBLE VITAMINS		
Vitamin A (retinyl palmitate)	1,500–5,000 IU	Long-term use of vitamin A (>10,000 IU) may increase bone loss in an aging population. Carotenoids, containing beta carotene, are vitamin A precursors that can be ingested in unlimited amounts. The body converts beta carotene to vitamin A on an as-needed basis. Carotenoids also contribute health benefits as antioxidants in their unconverted form as immune protectors and for cancer prevention.
Beta carotene and/or natural carotenoids (measured as vitamin A equivalencies)	10,000–25,000 IU	
Vitamin D (as calciferol)	200–400 IU	Some studies suggest 800 IU as chole-beneficial to protect bone. Aids calcium absorption. Conversion of vitamin D when exposed to sunlight most likely decreases with age.
Vitamin E (as d-alpha tocopheryl succinate or d-alpha tocopheryl acetate)	100–400 IU	Temporary boost to (3–6 months) 800–1200 IU for hot flash relief enhances immune system, relief of vaginal dryness, breast cysts and thyroid problems. Too much vitamin E can cause nausea, gas or diarrhea. Large amounts (>800 IU) taken for a prolonged time period may increase bleeding time.
Vitamin K OPTIONAL	20–400 mcg	
WATER-SOLUBLE VITAMINS		
Vitamin C (as ascorbic acid)	200–1,200 mg	

VITAMINS AND MINERALS WITH ESTABLISHED RECOMMENDED DAILY INTAKES (RDI)	AMOUNT PER SERVING RANGE MG/IU	WHAT YOU SHOULD KNOW
B-COMPLEX VITAMINS		
		Members of the B-complex vitamin family are water-soluble vitamins. They are washed away daily and are an aid to mood, mind, memory and liver metabolism.
B_1 (as thiamine mononitrate)	15–50 mg	Vitamin B_1 (thiamine) aids conversion of protein, carbohydrate and fat into energy, detoxification, heart and nervous systems. A shortage results in fatigue, depressions, "pins and needles" sensations or numbness in the legs.
B_2 (as riboflavin	15–50 mg	Vitamin B_2 (riboflavin) aids cellular energy, hormone production, neurotransmitter function, healthy eyes and skin and production of red blood cells.
B_3 (as a combination of niacin and niacinamide and not more than 10 mg niacin per day to reduce) experience of flushing)	50–500 mg	Niacin is important for release of energy from carbohydrates and the breakdown of fats and proteins. Niacin <10 mg per daily dose, otherwise can cause flushing. Niacinamide does not cause flushing, and it's beneficial for joint mobility.
Pantothenic acid	100–500 mg	Improves cholesterol synthesis; participates in hormone synthesis
Vitamin B_6 (as pyridoxine hydrochloride)	20–100 mg	Vitamin B_6 (pyridoxine) is helpful in protein synthesis, manufacture of hormones, red blood cells and over sixty enzymes and immune system function. Deficiency can result in a shortage of serotonin and contribute to depression.
Folate	200–800 mcg	Folic acid/folate deficiency is credited in 30 percent of coronary heart disease, blood vessel disease and strokes. Regulates cell division and supports healthy gums, red blood cells, gastrointestinal tract, immune system and central nervous system. Alleviates depression in the elderly and protects against Alzheimer's.
Vitamin B_{12}	100–1,000 mcg	Integral to a healthy nervous system; essential in the development of blood cells

VITAMINS AND MINERALS WITH ESTABLISHED RECOMMENDED DAILY INTAKES (RDI)	AMOUNT PER SERVING RANGE MG/IU	WHAT YOU SHOULD KNOW
Biotin	50–500 mcg	Healthy hair and nails
Choline (as choline bitartrate)	50–500 mg	Improves fat metabolism
Inositol	50–500 mg	Inositol aids nerve transmission and fat metabolism and can help relieve depression
Para-amino benzoic acid (PABA)	10–50 mg	
MINERALS		
Calcium (as any one or	250–500 mg	Avoid calcium carbonate or oyster shell calcium as the sole source of calcium. These forms of calcium neutralize stomach acid and have the potential to negatively impact digestion and the absorption of calcium. Oyster/coral shell can be contaminated. More on calcium selection below.
Magnesium (as any one or combination of glycinate, gluconate, citrate or oxide)	250–500 mg	Magnesium in the form of citrate acts as a laxative above 400 mg a day. Magnesium oxide is poorly utilized when combined with calcium carbonate. If a multimineral formula or magnesium product uses the oxide or citrate forms, then be certain they are combined with other delivery systems; for example, a combination of glycinate, citrate and oxide. Involved in over three hundred enzymatic reactions, including energy production. A deficiency intensifies reactions to stress by increasing the release of stress hormones.
Potassium (as aspartate)	50–99 mg	
Iron (as glycinate, citrate or fumarate)	5–10 mg	Iron becomes less important after menopause and should not be taken in a supplement because it could increase heart risks.
Zinc (as aspartate, gluconate, citrate)	10–20 mg	All minerals are attached to carriers. The significance of carriers is controversial. Choose minerals attached to carriers that are known to absorb well and not affect stomach acid pH balance. Mineral carriers derived from vegetable protein, or individual amino acids are excellent. Other
Manganese (as aspartate, gluconate, glycinate)	1–2 mg	
Copper (as lysinate, amino acid chelate)	1–2 mg	

VITAMINS AND MINERALS WITH ESTABLISHED RECOMMENDED DAILY INTAKES (RDI)	AMOUNT PER SERVING RANGE MG/IU	WHAT YOU SHOULD KNOW
Chromium (as cotinate glycinate or other amino acid carrier)	100–400 mcg	carriers are organic or inorganic salts dini- (calcium citrate, calcium carbonate). "Elemental mineral level" describes how much mineral is present.
Selenium (as aspartate or methionate)	100–400 mcg	Minerals are parts of enzymes and amino acids whose deficiencies can contribute to a number of diseases
Iodine (as potassium iodide)	50–200 mcg	whereas high doses of some, like iron, for example, can be toxic. Read below for details.
Molybdenum OPTIONAL	50–100 mcg	
Vanadium (as vanadyl sulfate) OPTIONAL	25–200 mcg	
Boron (as citrate) OPTIONAL	100–400 mcg	
NONESSENTIAL INGREDIENTS		
Avoid multivitamins/ minerals with herbal bases or herb extracts. (They introduce the possibility of allergenicity and adulter- ation; their levels are gener- ally too insignificant to be therapeutic.)		Herbs, enzymes, antioxidants, metabolites and isolated substances for which a specific individual amount is listed are placed below essential ingredients. When purchasing a multivitamin/mineral product, additional ingredients listed in this area can increase the cost and provide lim- ited health benefits because the levels are so low that they are considered insignificant from a health benefit perspective. Consider these ingredients to be merely "label dressing." They are probably valuable, BUT only when taken separately in the appro- priate form and correct amounts.

AFTER LABEL AND DOSAGE...THE REST OF THE STORY

In June of 2002, the *Journal of the American Medical Association* (*JAMA*) reversed its twenty-year antivitamin stance, recommending that daily supplementation is a good thing. Ultimately, it is not what you take, it is what you absorb that counts; this is called bioavailability. You want your vitamin pill to break down within thirty minutes and mix with whatever food you are eating.

Insure adequate amounts by not purchasing multivitamins you take once a day. They generally provide *minimal* amounts of supplements to prevent disease but do not augment organ and gland function or fortify reserves and strengthen the body's defenses. If you take a this type of multivitamin, follow directions carefully; extra pills can result in too much vitamin A or D.

To improve tolerance, make sure that common allergens such as yeast, soy, milk, egg, wheat, corn or artificial colorings are excluded. The label will give you dosage; a reputable company will keep within safe dosage. Avoid "mega-vitamins" that promise the moon but exceed safe limits and are less likely to have proper ratios between ingredients.

Select a multivitamin that includes a B-complex well in excess of the RDI (recommended daily dose). Look for a wide variety of antioxidants: natural-source carotenoids, lycopene, lutein, alpha carotene, cryptoxanthin, zeaxanthin and bioflavonoids such as quercetin and hesperiden.

Did you know**?** HRT depletes vitamin B_6, vitamin C, folic acid and niacin. Thyroid hormone depletes calcium. Antidepressants deplete melatonin. Blood pressure medications deplete potassium, magnesium and B vitamins. Oral antidiabetic agents deplete folic acid and B_{12}. Birth control pills deplete B vitamins.

In addition to your multivitamin, you will need to purchase a separate calcium supplement unless your multivitamin supplies a total of 1,000 mg in two or more doses per day. Do not waste your money on mega-doses. A midlife woman needs around 1,500 mg of calcium daily (800–1,000 mg before age fifty). The 1 percent of calcium not involved in building and strengthening bones and teeth insures that your muscles contract correctly, that your blood will clot and that nerves transport messages throughout your body. Depletion results in everything from insomnia, muscle cramps, agitation and depression, in addition to bone loss. If you do not consume enough calcium, your body will rob your bones to insure it gets what it needs for these vital processes.

As is true of vitamins and minerals, food remains an important source of calcium, but many women cut out calcium-rich foods from their diet. This comes back to haunt them as they age, especially if they did not get adequate amounts during rapid bone-building time in their teens. Caffeine and soft drinks deplete calcium, as well as too much milk or sugar, excess fat, protein, fiber or alcohol. Medications like tetracycline, corticosteroids, antacids, seda-tives, antibiotics and muscle relaxants also deplete calcium. If you are "burpy" or gassy after meals, take calcium with breakfast; otherwise, calcium at night will help you sleep and reduce leg cramps.

Use calcium carbonate when you need an antacid, but don't choose it as your best source of calcium. Calcium citrate is a better choice because it is well absorbed and slows bone loss. The "Cadillac" calcium is MCHC, or microcrystalline hydroxyapatite, a chemically complex raw bone concen-trate. MCHC promotes bone remineralization in postmenopausal women. MCHC is a complete bone food containing naturally occurring calcium along with a spectrum of ultra-trace minerals embedded in biologically active protein, which contains all that is needed to build bone.

Think about *it* . . . A study comparing absorp-tion of MCHC with calcium carbonate revealed MCHC was twice as effective in maintaining bone in postmenopausal osteoporotic women.[1]

IDENTIFYING ESSENTIAL OILS—OMEGA-3 FATTY ACIDS OR EPA/DHA SUPPLEMENTS YOU CAN TRUST

Increasing scientific evidence demonstrates that eicosapentaenoic acid (EPA) and docosahexaenoic acid (DHA), which your body does not make, powerfully influence cell membrane structure, composition and function. They benefit skin along with cardiovascular, central nervous system and retinal health. You must get them from food or supplements.

An EPA/DHA supplement insures proper hormone receptor function by either increasing or decreasing hormonal effects. If you supplement with "fish oil," quality is essential. The best choice for optimal absorption supplies EPA/DHA in triglyceride form. Buy from a company whose product is phar-maceutical grade and that guarantees it contains no harmful levels of mercury.

Other good sources of omega-3 come from flaxseed. Fresh ground organic flaxseed is preferred over the oil, but both are particularly helpful with hot flashes. The seeds provide both oil and flax fibers. The fibers are con-sumed by friendly bacteria in your colon and transformed into weak, but very beneficial, phytoSERMs. Should you wish to purchase flaxseed oil, we recom-mend Barlean's Flax Oil. The best way to use flax oil is as a salad dressing.

identifying essential oils you can trust

ESSENTIAL OILS	AMOUNT PER SERVING RANGE	WHAT YOU SHOULD KNOW
Natural marine lipid concentrate, enteric coated	1 gram	Look for supplements with enteric coating, which prevents repeating of fish oil taste and burping. If the label does not state the form of fish oil or guarantee freshness and purity, don't buy it.
EPA (eicosapentaenoic acid)	180–300 mg	Buying the concentrated oil is convenient and economical; 900 mg–1.5 grams of EPA daily.
DHA (docosahexaenoic acid)	120–200 mg	

IDENTIFYING PHYTOSERMS YOU CAN TRUST

A full-spectrum isoflavone concentrate from soy should have at its base a nongenetically modified (non-GMO) soy source. A finished third-party assay verifying label claim (amounts of total isoflavones and individual components) is essential to establish a meaningful dose.

identifying phytoSERMs you can trust

PHYTOSERMS	AMOUNT PER SERVING RANGE	WHAT YOU SHOULD KNOW
Soybean concentrate	100–350 mg	Beneficial Dose: 40–200 mg measured as total isoflavones daily
Total isoflavones containing:	40–100 mg	
Genistin/genistein (all forms)	20–50 mg	Amounts of genistin/genistein and daidzin/daidzein compounds that make up the phytoSERM portion of the total isoflavones should be present in approximately equal amounts, favoring more genistin/genistein
Daidzin/daidzein (all forms)	20–50 mg	
Glycitin/glycitein (all forms)	2–5 mg	

Consider *this...* The most expensive supplement is one that doesn't work or that you don't take.

A phytoestrogen molecule looks much like a human estrogen. They are classified into three groups and vary in their activity:

1. **Isoflavones** (genistin/genistein, daidzin/daidzein, glycitin/ glycitein, formononetin, biochanin A), found in soy and garbanzo beans and other legumes (tempeh, soy, miso, tofu, kudzu root, red clover), are hormonal regulators, weak estrogen mimics, antiestrogen, antioxidant and anticancer interventions. The amounts and ratios of actives vary from plant to plant.

2. **Lignans** are found in the cell walls of plants and are made bioavailable by the action of intestinal bacteria on grains (flaxseed, whole cereals like rye and wheat berries, brans and soybeans). They are hormonally active and known for their anticancer activity.

3. **Coumestans** are not a major natural source of phytoestrogens for humans (clover, sunflower seeds and bean sprouts).

Most American women consume less than 3 mg of isoflavones per day compared to Asian women, whose soy-based diet contains 40–80 mg per day. Higher isoflavone intake increases sex-hormone-binding globulin and, in conjunction with other chemical processes, lowers estrogen production.[2] This is particularly true in populations that have used them for a lifetime and less certain for those who increase their intake at a later age.

Still, new research suggests that consumption of as little as 10 mg per day may be associated with health benefits.[3] The genistein in soy increases the activity of dopamine and other neurotransmitters helpful for depression. Small studies have demonstrated relief of hot flashes by eating soy foods.[4] Others have confirmed the efficacy of soy extracts for hot flash relief.[5] Still other research studies report relief of vaginal dryness.[6] Soy foods are generally recommended over highly concentrated soy pills, especially for cancer patients, because supplement production changes the effect. However, women are not always good about adding tofu and the like to their diet. It really does not matter whether you consume fermented soy foods, such as tempeh, or nonfermented, such as tofu, because fermentation occurs through the action of gut bacteria. Genistin and daidzin are more prevalent in nonfermented soy.

What counts in the soybean concentrate you purchase, fermented or nonfermented, is the actual amount of isoflavones on the label—verified by independent third-party analysis.

Caution: Too much soy is known to decrease thyroid function and to deactivate thyroid medication.

SOY SENSITIVE OR ALLERGIC?

If you suspect an allergic reaction to soy, consider red clover, kudzu or garbanzo beans, etc.

if soy sensitive or allergic, try...

Red clover flowering top extract (*Trifolium pretense*)	Cancer-protective capacity.[7] Contains isoflavones, formononetin and biochanin A, shown to bind to estrogen receptors and to produce estrogen-like effects.[8] Hot flash relief, increases high density lipoprotein levels (HDL) but unlike estrogen does not cause changes in uterine thickness.
Kudzu root extract (*Pueraria lobata*)	New source of isoflavones. Used traditionally to support heart and liver function.
Total isoflavone content from either one or a combination of both plants should provide 40–100 mg. The amounts of genistein, daidzein and additional isoflavones should be disclosed on label.	

A PERSONAL TESTIMONY

Throughout *Good for You!* I have complained of my struggle with hot flashes. I am aware of the lifestyle factors that are contributing to their intensity and my personal health issues that disrupt my thermoregulatory system. It was frustrating to find that many of the natural products that worked so well for everyone else were less effective for me. However, I have persevered and am pleased to share that even I have found considerable relief (and quickly) from a product that has a base of red clover. After several weeks on the suggested dose, I was able to reduce the number of pills and still obtain relief. I have included the ingredients in the discussion that follows because it is a good example of what you will increasingly see in the marketplace—a natural foundational combination product designed to cover many of the bases HRT was thought to cover. There is, however, no comparison in the risk/benefit ratio between HRT and this natural product. Symptom relief that improves my health without risk is the best of all worlds.

A NEW ERA IN WOMEN'S PRODUCTS: CHOOSING A MULTIFUNCTIONAL FORMULA

What follows is an example of a multifunctional approach to balancing estrogen positively while supporting detoxification. The formula combines non-soy isoflavones, phytonutrients, antioxidants, select vitamins and a blend of active folates. The combination addresses multiple factors related to estrogen, without adding estrogen hormone. It seeks to balance and maximize endogenous estrogen and to use the adaptogen abilities of phytoestrogens to relieve symptoms and protect against the bad-girl forms of estrogen. This is one of the first examples of innovative products that you will likely see more of as a replacement for HRT.

When this supplement was tested in a pilot study on women who had severe hot flashes and night sweats, there was a 46 percent drop in hot flashes and a similar improvement in quality of life scores as measured by a standardized menopause quality of life questionnaire. Additionally, there was modest improvement in cholesterol/HDL ratios and homocysteine. A marker of breast cancer risk (2-OH/16-OH ratio) showed a statistically significant improvement.[9] It is encouraging, and one would hope increasingly more common, to see a natural medicine company put time and money into a well-designed clinical trial for menopause, substantiating their claims and publishing their research. (See chart below for specifics.)

ESTROFACTORS

Below is a label of supplement facts from a product called EstroFactors. This product can be purchased from many natural practitioners, physicians or Metagenics. It is also available on our Web site. As you are looking at the label, please note the following:

> **[A]** Vitamin E is correlated with elevated estrogen levels; it increases detoxification with A and protects immune function.
>
> **[B]** D regulates absorption of calcium and phosphorous; along with vitamin K, it aids in normal blood clotting and bone strength.
>
> **[C]** Folates, along with B vitamins, aid in stress relief, PMS symptom reduction, detoxification; homocysteine metabolism is aided by L-5MTHF to insure proper folate utilization.

[D] Chrysin is a bioflavonoid and may inhibit cell-proliferation of estrogen.

[E] PhytoSERMs: Non-soy isoflavones provide daidzein, genistein, puerarin and for-monetin.

[F] Rosemary enhances 2-OH estrogen metabolite production and helps detoxifica-tion. Turmeric may protect tissue from reactive estrogen metabolites.

[G] Resveratrol is an estrogen agonist and antagonist.

Supplement Facts

	Amount Per Day (in three tablets)
Vitamin A (50 percent as betatene mixed carotenoids and 50 percent as retinyl palmitate)	2,500 IU
Vitamin E (as d-alpha tocopheryl acetate) (see [A])	200 IU
Vitamin D (as cholecalciferol) (see [B])	200 IU
Vitamin K	40 mcg
Folate* (L-5 methyl tetrahydrofolate†, folic acid and 5-formyl tetrahydrofolate) (see [C])	800 mcg
B_{12} (as methylcobalamin and cyanocobalamin) 30 mcg	
Trimethylglycine	200 mg
Chrysin (see [D])	90 mg
Isoflavones (from a proprietary blend of red clover blossoms *(Trifolium pretense)* and kudzu root extract *(Pueraria lobata)*	100 mg**
Turmeric rhizome extract *(Curcuma longa)* standardized to 95 percent curcuminoids	210 mg**
Rosemary leaf extract *(Rosmarinus offcinalis)* contains not less than 5.1 percent carnosic acid and carnosol (see [F])	200 mg**
Resveratrol (from *Polygonum cuspidatum*) (see [G])	2 mg**

† As Metafollin U.S. Patent Nos. 5,997,915; 6,254,904. Patent Pending
*Featuring ActiFolate: a proprietary blend of active folates
** Daily value not established

I must emphasize that relief for my hot flashes did not come with the first natural product I tried or even as a result of my good supplement regimen. It may not for you, either. Remember, you are a scientist. When you have eliminated what doesn't work, you still may not draw conclusions about whether any natural product will ever work for you. Keep reading; make sure your foundational nutrition is in order. Are your vitamins good quality? Is your fish oil supplement the right kind? Have you increased the phytoSERMs in your diet? You may need more. If so, read on. Natural relief for specific symptoms and groups of symptoms will be discussed in the next chapter.

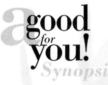

1. What would it take to motivate you to make optimizing your health and adopting a foundational supplement plan a priority? What gets in your way?

2. If your symptoms aren't relieved at a level you desire, are you willing to keep up the scientific pursuit of something with a low risk profile or will you go back on HRT?

3. Are you concerned about influencing your estrogen to be a "good girl" and protecting yourself from degenerative diseases of aging, or do you just want the symptoms to go away?

14

i will do this much: natural relief

The foundational supplement program outlined in chapter thirteen is an effective beginning point, capable of providing many women all they need to relieve symptoms of aging or menopause while supplying protection against disease and increasing energy. If you have concluded that the supplements you are currently taking are of mediocre quality, take the challenge to find others that are good. They may provide the relief you need. And remember, feeling better is also dependent on how sturdy the three legs of your foundation are: nutrition, exercise and stress management.

Give yourself four to eight weeks on the foundational supplement program, and then reevaluate your symptoms. You may see some change sooner—sometimes within the first seven days. If your changes seem insignificant or transient, make sure you are taking your foundation program every day. If you are, you may need to increase your dose within the acceptable upper ranges. Even then, some may find more is needed.

This chapter will provide further options depending on the particular group of symptoms that are most annoying or distressing. We recommend that you select one supplement from the additional intervention list that best addresses core complaints and add it to your foundation supplement support. This will reinforce the action of the foundation program and hopefully speed up response. Be sure to adjust the amounts of supplements you are currently taking to achieve beneficial supplement levels recommended in the box.

Even though several choices are suggested, we are not recommending you try each one. Such an all-encompassing approach isn't necessarily better and is sure to be expensive. Some choices will fit your lifestyle and personality more than others. Some simply won't work for you—or won't work quickly enough. There is a point when it may be appropriate to seek professional support from an expert in the area of natural, functional or traditional medicine.

NATURAL RELIEF: TELL ME WHAT TO DO

If you have symptoms that you want to get rid of, this chapter is where the rubber meets the road. It does not contain suggestions for some of the chronic diseases of aging; those will be discussed in chapter sixteen. There is a spill-over effect, however. The worst thing that can happen as you introduce these interventions is that you will be healthier.

Of course, you have many choices. You can choose to ignore looking at the big picture and concentrate on the immediate—a quick-fix approach. You can choose an herbal product without consideration of the diagnostics mentioned in chapter eight or the foundational supplements of the last chapter. If symptoms are bad enough and/or don't respond quickly enough, you can go back on HRT. You can keep reading and decide to do more if "I will only do this much" does not bring you the relief you need. You can do everything or part of—as you struggle with voices that say, "Nothing will help."

It is a reality, however, that you can manage symptoms safely. And you must start somewhere. For those who love charting and detailed order, keep a calendar for a month on which you mark the severity (mild, moderate, severe) for various menopause or aging concerns. Or better yet, fill out the Women's Health Questionnaire (WHQ) in Appendix C. Filling out the WHQ has the advantage of providing a means of objectively determining how effective your intervention has been.

For the more free-flowing amongst us, sit down, get yourself a cup of tea and give a few minutes thought to the symptoms that are your greatest concern or most bothersome. Even if you are asymptomatic, you still need foundational support as outlined in the previous chapter.

MIDLIFE ANGST: I WANT TO GET RID OF, REDUCE...

Today it is possible to go into a store and purchase potato chips that claim to enhance memory, New Age drinks that promise vitality and candy that reduces hot flashes. Even if the nutrients in these products reached a "clinically effective level," the transfatty acids, sugar and calories would do you in. We have to advise you to leave such choices on the shelf and choose, instead, foods containing naturally occurring phytochemicals.

On the other hand, natural products and supplements prepared in doses that have been shown to be "clinically effective" and "standardized" for greatest efficacy (rather than snacking) can powerfully modify biological function. The natural choices that Lyra and I are suggesting are ones that have the highest degree of clinical support. Some have been used traditionally for generations and are only now being accepted in our culture as viable clinical options as investigators uncover the biochemical reasons for why they work.

We have included a variety of approaches to healing because not every course will be the best for you. Unlike a prescription medication, you can risk experimenting within the parameters of what has been deemed suitable dosage. A little trial and error is appropriate and may be essential. You may need to change the time of day you take a product or whether or not you take it with food.

The botanicals and mixtures reviewed in this chapter promote balance within glandular and organ systems challenged by stress, lifestyle and diet to alleviate menopausal symptoms. Commercial availability, quality, safety, appropriate dosage form and ability to deliver reasonable efficacy are the five pivotal criteria used to determine which herbs and formulas were included.

Determining the symptom pattern that characterizes your midlife complaints is your first step. Again, we encourage you to use the WHQ as your baseline. It will help you more easily determine how successful your foundation program is and, based on the intensity and frequency of your symptom pattern, whether or not you want to add an additional supplement. The second challenge is sorting through the variety of forms these products come in and selecting the gems that are right for you. We will give you specific guidelines to follow.

your natural relief options

Black cohosh root and rhizome • St. John's wort flowering tops • Chasteberry fruit and seed • Ginkgo leaf • Nature-identical progesterone • Dehydroepiandosterone (DHEA) • Ginseng root • Classic ancient traditional Chinese herbal formula • A joint and connective tissue specific remedy

NATURAL HELP FOR HOT/COLD FLASHES...AND MORE!

You probably don't need help in determining how problematic hot/cold flashes are! They run the gamut from mildly irritating to nearly debilitating. Relief comes through a variety of actions and interventions. It is helpful to note when hot flashes are most apt to occur. Are you upset? Stressed? Is it the same time of day? Is there a pattern? It is confusing when the ebb and flow of hormones during the transition from menstruating to cessation of menses seesaws between periods of hormone stability and a dramatic drop in estrogen, announced with an onslaught of hot flashes and sweats.

This constant flux makes it important to adjust the amount and frequency of supplements you take as well as black cohosh. Find the lowest amount that works. This gives you the opportunity to increase the amount as needed.

Do not underestimate taking care of the obvious: keep rooms cool, use absorbent fabrics and sheets, and avoid confining and heavy clothing, hot drinks, alcohol, caffeine, chocolate, soft drinks, sugar and spicy foods. Don't exercise or take a hot bath right before bedtime. Exercise, however, can be very effective in reducing hot flashes. Deep abdominal breathing works—as long as you begin to breathe deeply at the onset of symptoms.

Those vegetarians who are careful with their protein levels have fewer hot flashes, so mimic them and eat your broccoli. Be aware that hot flashes are interrelated with thyroid and adrenal function, so if the interventions mentioned don't bring you relief, you may need to consider some of the suggestions in the next chapter.

In the following chart, check symptoms or behaviors that occur throughout the month with a frequency or intensity that affects your daily activities or your ability to feel good about yourself.

my menopausal symptoms

❑	1.	Decline of energy/sense of well-being	❑	8.	Vaginal problems
			❑	9.	Joint and muscle pain
❑	2.	Hot flashes	❑	10.	Change in sexual desire
❑	3.	Night sweats	❑	11.	Loss of muscle tone
❑	4.	Spontaneous sweating	❑	12.	Fatigue; dragging, tired feeling
❑	5.	Chills	❑	13.	Weight gain
❑	6.	Depression	❑	14.	Fluid retention
❑	7.	Urinary problems	❑	15.	Difficulty concentrating

Did you check one or more menopausal symptoms in addition to hot flashes? What did your WHQ reveal?

About black cohosh

Black cohosh roots and rhizomes *(Actaea racemosa syn Cimicifuga racemosa)* were used by Native American tribes living on the eastern parts of the United States. The traditional application inspired research for menopausal symptoms. Several decades of study are currently available that demonstrate black cohosh extract can positively impact hot flashes and mood swings. Currently, black cohosh alone and in combination with other natural ingredients is the most widely used plant for perimenopausal symptoms in the U.S. and Europe.

The most extensively investigated commercial form of black cohosh is Remifemin. This is a proprietary form, but by no means the only or most effective option. A black cohosh product combined with complementary herbs or additional B vitamins is a good, often economical, option. Remember to insure you are purchasing a good product by recalling the criteria from chapter twelve.

The Complete German Commission E Monographs states that "black cohosh has estrogen-like actions, suppresses luteinizing hormone, binds to estrogen receptors, and has no contraindications to its use, with occasional gastric discomfort as the only side effect."[1] In 2003, the North American Menopause Society essentially came to the same conclusion after an extensive literature review.[2] It is important to understand that black cohosh is not an estrogen or phytoSERM, but a hormone-regulating herb that seems to affect the hypothalamus, pituitary gland and estrogen receptors. It does not promote endometrial growth like estrogen does. It should not be used with HRT, although several studies have combined it with Tamoxifen. The daily effective dose depends on the form of black cohosh that you take. We recommend taking 160 mg per day of the specific kind of standardized extract.

The following chart shows the information to look for on your label of black cohosh supplement:

Supplement Facts

	Amount Per Day Range
Standardized Extract	
Black cohosh root and rhizome extract (*Actaea racemosa*, also called *Cimicifuga racemosa*) standardized to 2.5 percent triterpene glycosides expressed as 27-deoxyactein and other naturally occurring terpene	80–160 mg

Crude Extract

Black cohosh root and rhizome (*Actaea racemosa*, also called *Cimicifuga racemosa*) crude extracts where the recommended dose will provide levels close to 2.5 percent triterpene glycosides

Daily serving varies with the composition or concentration ratio of crude extract. Do not use if the information is not available.

Powdered Root (not an extract)

Black cohosh root and rhizome (*Actaea racemosa*, also called *Cimicifuga racemosa*) powder   1,000–2,000 mg

A summary of options for hot/cold flashes

Along with the options summarized in the following chart, revisit your foundational use of vitamin E and EPA/DHA.

hot/cold flash options

OPTIONS	FORM AND DOSAGE	SIDE EFFECTS	TIME FOR EFFICACY	SERENDIPITY
Black cohosh (*Cimicifuga Actaea racimosa syn racemosa*)	Powder: 1–2 grams Tea: 1–2 grams 3 x day Fluid extract: 1 teaspoon (1:1) or 250–500 Standardized extract: 80–160 mg/day	Very low incidence of temporary mild gastrointestinal upset	Two weeks to four months	Vaginal lubrication and help with depression, mild pain relief
Black cohosh combines well with vitamin E, B vitamins, calcium, magnesium, St. John's wort flowering tops *(Hypericum perforatum)*, sources of isoflavones, some traditional herbs such as motherwort herb *(Leonurus cardiaca)*, lemon balm herb *(Melissa officinalis)*. Reputable medical herb companies combine herbs consistent with herbal traditions. Remember, to insure clinical benefits consistent with clinical trials, there MUST be the significant levels of black cohosh in the recommended daily dose.				
Deep breathing	Abdominal breaths[3]	None	Immediate if caught in time	Stress level is reduced, energized, improved mood, mental capacity
Accupressure	With left hand, press between eyebrows or backside of shoulder	None	Immediate	No cost, no equipment!
Acupuncture[4]	Practitioner required/eight sessions	None	87 percent; relief one month later	Tested with women with breast cancer using Tamoxifen physical and emotional well-being benefited, better sleep

BLEEDING IRREGULARITIES AND/OR PREMENSTRUAL SYNDROME

It is difficult to distinguish between irregular bleeding caused by menopausal shutdown or from other causes that can require a physician's attention. Erratic bleeding may be light, heavy or occur apart from the normal time of the period. Always take such incidents seriously, and consult your doctor. Vaginal sonography (ultrasound) is less invasive than other procedures that might be used to determine whether observation is in order or a more active intervention is called for.

---

hormonal and ovarian imbalance

Check symptoms or behaviors that occur throughout the month with a frequency or intensity that affects your daily activities or your ability to feel good about yourself.

❑ Anxiety
❑ Irritability
❑ Temporary weight gain
❑ Water retention
❑ Abdominal bloating
❑ Tender/swollen breasts
❑ Craving for sweets

❑ Heart palpitations
❑ Depression
❑ Heavy prolonged periods
❑ Unusually light periods
❑ Irregular periods
❑ Bleeding or spotting between periods

While perimenopausal bleeding can be scary, its origin is explainable. As ovarian function declines, ovulation is irregular, expressed as missed periods and breakthrough bleeding. This means less progesterone is produced to balance estrogen. It is why you may have heard people speak of menopause being a state of estrogen dominance as opposed to estrogen insufficiency. The lining of the uterus (endometrium) is primed by estrogen (proliferative effect) to thicken it, and it can slough off irregularly, causing heavy bleeding during and between cycles.

Chasteberry *(Vitex agnus-castus)*

Chasteberry is believed to cause longer healthy ovulation, therefore elongated exposure to endogenous progesterone and more normal cycles.

It is a surprise sometimes to find a new surge or intensified premenstrual syndrome (PMS) rearing its annoying head at midlife. It is not uncommon for PMS to worsen as menopause approaches whether or not it has been an issue during a woman's reproductive years. Moodiness, bloating, sugar cravings around the period or the time the period used to be can be a concern. Chasteberry is also helpful for hormonal imbalance that expresses itself as PMS and dysfunctional uterine bleeding. (Refer to parts one and three of the WHQ.)

About chasteberry

Chasteberry has a hormone-like action enabling it to bind with estrogen receptors. It was used by Greek physicians to regulate female menstrual cycles almost two thousand years ago. It aids vaginal dryness and appears to encourage balanced progesterone synthesis by supporting healthy uterine lining and ovarian function.[5]

The following chart shows what to look for on a label for chasteberry.

Supplement Facts

	Amount Per Day Range
Chasteberry Fruit 10:1 Extract *(Vitex agnus-castus)*	100–200 mg
Chasteberry Fruit Powder *(Vitex agnus-castus)*	500–1,000 mg
Agnolyt Liquid (proprietary preparation of *Vitex*)	As directed

A summary of options for PMS and bleeding irregularities

Along with the suggestions from the following chart, revisit your foundational use of fish oils, B complex, vitamin C and calcium/magnesium. Also consider using evening primrose oil for symptomatic relief of PMS.

PMS and bleeding irregularity options

OPTIONS	FORM AND DOSAGE	SIDE EFFECTS	TIME FOR EFFICACY	SERENDIPITY
Chasteberry *(Vitex agnus-castus)*	100–200 mg capsule or tablet per day of crude 10:1 extract	Decreases libido in men, increases in women	One to three months	PMS relief, vaginal lubrication, normal menses
Evening primrose oil as source of omega-6 fatty acids	300–450 mg as GLA	Skin rash, headache; do not take if prone to seizures, blood clots	One to three months	Healthy hair, skin and nails; elevated mood

The following chart shows what to look for on a label for evening prim-rose oil.

Supplement Facts

	Amount Per Capsule Range
Evening Primrose Oil	
Supplying Gamma-Linoleic Acid (GLA) and	50–100 mg
Linoleic Acid (LA)	360–750 mg

DRYNESS VAGINALLY/TRIPS TO THE BATHROOM

As estrogen production wanes, its tissue-building ability is reduced. The vulva and vaginal area (including the urethra) become thinner and frailer. There is an increased chance for small vaginal tears that not only increase the possibility of infection but also result in painful intercourse. Anything that decreases dryness overall can be helpful and may or may not resolve the issue. Avoid dyes, perfumes and synthetic underwear that can further irri-tate fragile tissue.

dryness

Check symptoms or behaviors that occur throughout the month with a frequency or intensity that affects your daily activities or your ability to feel good about yourself.

- ❑ Vaginal itching, burning, dryness
- ❑ Abnormal vaginal discharge
- ❑ Frequent urination
- ❑ Painful intercourse
- ❑ Dry skin, hair, nails

This breakdown also results in increased trips to the bathroom—the tis-sues involved are all embryonically related and therefore equally affected. Losing weight is sometimes helpful. The University of San Francisco reported that urinary incontinence decreased by 53 percent following a three-month weight loss program.[6] Many women find vaginal dryness and urinary incontinence are not easily resolved, especially after discontinuing hormone replacement. Do not ignore the condition in hopes it will improve on its own. If the interventions suggested here do not bring relief, consider those offered in the next chapter. If you continue to have multiple infections, increased itching and a need to urinate and/or painful intercourse, consult your physician.

Natural vitamin E and mixed tocopherols

Vitamin E counteracts dryness. While we are suggesting oral use, some women find relief by breaking open the capsule and applying the oil directly to the vaginal/urethral area.

The following chart shows what to look for on a label for vitamin E.

Supplement Facts

Soft gel capsules only	Amount Per Day Range
Vitamin E (as d-alpha tocopherol)	400–1,200 IU
Other naturally occurring tocopherols:	
Gamma tocopherol	270–850 mg
Delta tocopherol	90–270 mg
Beta tocopherol	5–15 mg

A SUMMARY OF OPTIONS FOR VAGINAL/URINARY PROBLEMS

Along with the suggestions offered in the following chart, revisit your foundational use of vitamin E and fish oils.

vaginal/urinary problem options

OPTIONS	FORM AND DOSAGE	SIDE EFFECTS	TIME FOR EFFICACY	SERENDIPITY
Natural vitamin E (mixed tocopherols with a standardized level of d-alpha tocopherol	Oral 400–800 IU as d-alpha tocopherol, applied as an oil to vagina	Blood thinner; diarrhea/gas with high doses. Don't use with high blood pressure, digitalis, diabetes, rheumatic heart disease; consult physician		Many benefits to heart, memory
Magnesium (citrate)	350 mg 2x day	Loose stools or diarrhea	Within one month; after two weeks dosage can be increased if needed	Relief of constipation, very inexpensive
Regular intercourse	"Use it or lose it" applies here by stimulating lubrication. Use a water-soluble lubricant EVERY time you make love (K-Y Lubricating Jelly, Astroglide or AquaLube), and apply moisturizers like Replens or Gyne-Moistrin for daily comfort.	Lubricants will go far in prevention and worsening this common condition		Women who have regular sexual relations enjoy sex more than those who have sex infrequently, and they feel better about their relationship.

SKIN/HAIR DRYNESS: THE WRINKLE CURE

A lack of estrogen results in a decrease of collagen—the main supportive protein of our entire body. I have heard more than one woman declare that she will stay on HRT for this very reason alone. With less collagen thickness there is increased wrinkling, drying, thinning, mutations in pigment and reduced elasticity. Skin can become "itchy" and sensitive to touch. Bruising is more likely because of greater vessel fragility. We urge you to consider other options with less of a risk/benefit trade-off if this is your sole reason for remaining on HRT. Dermatologists and the cosmetics industry offer an increasing array of products that actually do what they claim.

A summary of options for dry skin/wrinkles

Along with suggestions given in the following chart, revisit your foundational use of vitamin E, C, fish oils and evening primrose oil.

skin health options

OPTIONS	FORM AND DOSAGE	SIDE EFFECTS	TIME FOR EFFICACY	SERENDIPITY
Vitamin E complex	Look for in cosmetic products		Cosmetic product use can be in weeks	Many benefits for cardiovascular and neurological health
Vitamin C (pH balanced with minerals and antioxidants)	Orally: 1–3 grams; topically: cosmetic products	Too much vitamin C can cause loose stool	Cosmetic product use can be in weeks	Helps immune system; increases energy, neurotransmitters; reduces inflammation
Sunscreen* (A product recommended by dermatologists that absorbs quickly and doesn't run and sting the eyes is Ocean Potion (50) antiaging sunblock with UVA 1 and 2, UVB, Parsol 1789, vitamins A, C and E; more information at www.opotion.com)	30 SPF with protection from both UVA and UVB; use daily as you do moisturizers	There are new products that do not sting the eyes	Daily damage is decreased immediately	Some products have vitamin C; B complex included for skin repair; makeup generally is not high enough SPF rating
Alpha lipoic acid	Lotion or cream applied daily		Weeks	
DMAE dimethylaminoethanol	Lotion or cream applied daily		Weeks	Antioxidant membrane stabilizer
Alpha hydroxy and beta hydroxy acids	Lotion or cream applied daily	Can irritate sensitive skin	Weeks	Increases cell turnover
Water	8 glasses or more per day	None	Weeks	The "oil" that keeps the body running smoothly; increased weight loss; add lemon or herbs to lightly flavor; take it with you
Reduce stress	High stress results in blood being sent to vital organs and neglecting your skin	None	Immediate	Benefit to all systems; pleasure of life

onsider *this...* Studies have found an association between nutrients in your blood stream, your diet and the condition of your skin. Smooth skin starts from the inside.[7]

FATIGUE AND SLEEPLESSNESS

Most women today have a reason to be tired. It is the rare individual whose life is serene and balanced. Psychological and spiritual struggles that increase at midlife and as we age can contribute to fatigue. For many women, tiredness is due to interrupted sleep from hot flashes.

Medications frequently keep people awake. Check both over-the-counter and prescription drugs you are taking. Physical pain not only makes you restless, but it also increases cortisol and the fight-or-flight response. If no amount of restorative rest or sleep helps you feel rested, and especially if you are more tired thirty minutes after exercising than refreshed, a deeper problem is likely. Adrenal and thyroid imbalances are apt to be involved and should be addressed. (See chapters eleven and fifteen.) There are natural approaches that can help you restore restful sleep.

peri- and postmenopause

Check symptoms or behaviors that occur throughout the month with a frequency or intensity that affects your daily activities or your ability to feel good about yourself.

- ❑ Decline of energy/sense of well-being
- ❑ Hot flashes
- ❑ Night sweats
- ❑ Spontaneous sweating
- ❑ Chills
- ❑ Depressed
- ❑ Urinary problems

- ❑ Vaginal problems
- ❑ Joint and muscle pain
- ❑ Change in sexual desire
- ❑ Loss of muscle tone
- ❑ Fatigue; feeling tired, dragging
- ❑ Weight gain
- ❑ Fluid retention
- ❑ Difficulty concentrating

TRADITIONAL CHINESE MEDICINE (TCM)

Chinese medicine approaches to health are built around "balance." Vital energy, or Qi (pronounced *chee*), provides a gateway to an evaluation as to whether you are "in balance" (on a number of levels) and healthy or "out of balance" and unhealthy. Energy channels are known as *meridians*. Acupuncture and accupressure manipulate these meridians to rebalance energy flow through the insertion of needles (acupuncture), massage, heat and electro-stimulation of specific points that run in channels along the surface of the body. While meridians don't appear to follow neurological pathways, they do correspond to areas where connective tissues, which run throughout the body, are thickest.

Acupuncture is the most researched of all forms of TCM showing effective results particularly with pain relief, hot flashes and nausea. It boosts the levels of the body's own naturally produced painkillers (opiates known as endorphins) and increases serotonin, which improves mood.

Herb use is never of the "pill-for-an-ill" variety. Traditional Chinese botanical preparations are recommended based on the sign and symptom patterns expressed by the patient. They are designed to correct the fundamental imbalances underlying the symptoms. There are typical perimenopausal and menopausal clinical pictures common to many women the world over that respond to several classic botanical mixtures made up of what are called *adaptogenic plants*—plants that enhance the body's ability to adapt to stress. The traditional Chinese practitioners have no problem evaluating health from a functional perspective; they invariably look at the "big" picture.

ere you *wondering***?** An herbal *adaptogen* has a normalizing effect that does not influence body function more than required.

About ginseng

In traditional Chinese medicine (TCM), ginseng is one of the world's oldest herbal remedies and is the most valued and widely used herb in China and Asia. A major problem in recommending ginseng is the unreliability of its products. Look for standardized, high-quality extracts. Ginseng comes in many versions: Asian, Korean and Chinese are considered "true ginseng" (*Panax ginseng, Panax* meaning "cure all or panacea") and are categorized as "warming and stimulating." American ginseng (*Panax quinquefolium*) is different from the Asian species; it possesses "calming and cooling" properties and is therefore used differently. Confused with *Panax* are Siberian, Russian "ginseng" (*Eleuthrococcus senticosus*), which enhances physical and mental stamina, and Ashwagandha, Indian ginseng (*Withania somnifera*), which protects from physical and chemical stressors.

Ginseng is given most as an adaptogen. It is used differently in Asia than in Europe. For optimal results in menopause, we recommend using ginseng according to the ancient Chinese tradition. From both an Eastern and a Western perspective, ginseng has properties that normalize body functions, restoring the body's balance, enhancing stamina and increasing resistance to stress and disease. The difference between approaches surrounds the dose and the applications.

Western European applications frequently recommend too little plant to address acute or chronic health conditions. However, research on a proprietary extract, known as Ginsana, suggests that a dose of 100–200 mg of *Panax ginseng* root extract standardized to 4 percent ginsenosides (4–8 mg per day) was adequate to enhance stamina and performance. While it did not reduce hot flashes, it did help improve menopausal quality of life issues such as depression and well-being.[8] To get the most out of ginseng for menopause, review your menopause symptoms. Feeling cold and clammy versus hot, listless, depressed, apathetic and fatigued calls for ginseng. Choose a concentrated high-quality ginseng extract and take it at levels consistent with the recommendations listed in the following Supplement Facts box.

Supplement Facts

	Amount Per Day Range
Asian ginseng root extract *(Panax ginseng)* (standardized to 5–8% ginsenosides), supplying 40–80 mg ginsenosides of 5% extract or 64–128 mg ginsenosides of 8% extract	400–1,600 mg
Asian ginseng root powder *(Panax ginseng)*	1,000–4,000 mg

About Celestial Emperor's Heart Supplementing Elixir (Serenagen)

This wonderfully named elixir was first used in the Yuan Dynasty (1279–1368). While not researched in the West, the formula is widely used in China and among TCM practitioners internationally. Rehmannia root (*Rehmannia glutinosa* or sheng di haung) is a chief herb in the formula and is known for its ability to positively influence blood sugar in the liver, while protecting the liver itself, replenishing exhausted reserves and supporting the kidneys and the circulatory system. You can find this ancient product under the traditional name Tian Wang Bu Xin Dan or a variety of proprietary names such as Serenagen and Stress Rescue. Dong quai root (*Angelica sinensis*) also appears, used in combination with other support herbs, as it is traditionally used. Research that demonstrated dong quai's ineffectiveness for treating hot flashes used in dong quai as a sole ingredient.

The chart below shows what to look for on a label for Serenagen.

Supplement Facts

	Amount Per Tablet
Serenagen formula	500 mg
Prepared as a dried 5:1 water extract	
Rehmannia root (*Rehmannia glutinosa*) (see [A])	
Ginseng root *(Panax ginseng)* (see [B])	
Poria fungus *(Poria cocos)* (see [B])	
Dong quai root (*Angelica sinensis*) (see [C])	
Salvia root (*Salvia miltiorrhiza*) (see [C])	
Biota seed (*Biota orientals*) (see [D])	
Polygala root (*Polygala tenuifolia*) (see [D])	
Schizandra fruit (*Schizandra Chinese*) (see [E])	
Jujube fruit (*Zizyphus spinosa*) (see [E])	
Asparagus root (*Asparagus chochinchinensis*) (see [F])	
Ophiopogon root (*Ophiopogon japonicus*) (see [F])	
Scrophularia root (*Scrophularia ningpoensis*) (see [F])	
Platycodon root (Platycodon grandiflorum) (see [G])	

[A] Replenishes reserves; nourishes blood; balances blood sugar

[B] Enhances stamina, blood flow, oxygen transport, cardiac contractility

[C] Supports circulation/heart

[D] Sedative

[E] Supports oxygen transport

[F] Aids integrity of heart tissue and function

[G] Protects reserves, healthy detoxification

Choosing heart elixir depends on how hot, dry and irritated you feel. Since both ginseng and heart elixir address hot flashes and feelings of fatigue, the decision to take one or the other is based on how you feel most of the time. Their point of departure is around the general tenor of your emotions: irritable/dry–heart elixir or apathetic/waterlogged–ginseng.

Summary of options for fatigue and sleeplessness

In addition to the suggestions in the chart below, revisit your foundational use of vitamin B complex and vitamin E.

fatigue and sleeplessness options

OPTIONS	FORM AND DOSAGE	SIDE EFFECTS	TIME FOR EFFICACY	SERENDIPITY
Ginseng root	Ginseng root extract standardized to 5–8 percent ginsenosides: 400–1,600 mg/day; main root powder: 3–5 grams	Safe; during menopause, may cause breakthrough bleeding, tender breasts; lowers blood concentrations of alcohol and warfarin. Do not use with MAO inhibiting drugs for depression. Take with prescription medications only under supervision of CAM practitioner. Avoid if prone to hormone-related health problems.[9]	Allow four weeks	Increased stamina and energy; balancing of mood; blood sugar regulation; reduction in arrhythmias
TCM emperor's tea	3 grams of 5:1 extract daily	Very safe; do not use with prescription medications unless under supervision of CAM practitioner.	Allow two weeks	Balancing of mood; blood sugar regulation; reduction in arrhythmias and blood pressure; restful sleep
Water	8 glasses per day		Immediate	All systems function more efficiently
Exercise	Any—but walking is great, just not right before bedtime; minimally 10 minutes 3x per day	None		Beneficial to every system in the body, improves mood
Stabilize blood sugar	Low-glycemic food; small meals 6x per day; balanced bedtime snack			Weight loss

MEMORY AND CONCENTRATION: GINKGO BILOBA

There is nothing more distressing than thinking you are losing your mind. Changes in memory and concentration are noted at menopause because the hippocampus (learning and memory center) depends on estrogen to interact with its many estrogen receptors. The brain's neurotransmitters are influenced by estrogen. Inability to remember words and names of things can be a sign of estrogen in short supply. Most of the changes in memory, however, are normal changes of aging, and many are due to our failure to give adequate attention to learning something in the first place. Clear thinking can be affected by inadequate blood sugar levels and atherosclerotic plaque, which can prevent blood from getting to the brain (foggy brain). There are many physical and medication-induced causes of memory problems; check with your doctor.

memory/concentration changes

Check symptoms or behaviors that occur throughout the month with a frequency or intensity that affects your daily activities or your ability to feel good about yourself.

- ❑ Difficulty absorbing new information
- ❑ Easily distracted
- ❑ Tendency to become frustrated
- ❑ Agitation/inability to sit still
- ❑ Confusion
- ❑ Depression
- ❑ Irritability
- ❑ Anxiety
- ❑ Mood swings
- ❑ Headaches
- ❑ Forgetfulness
- ❑ Difficulty concentrating
- ❑ Difficulty sleeping

About ginkgo

The use of ginkgo is recorded in ancient Chinese medical texts dating back twenty-eight hundred years. It is the oldest living tree species. One of the safest herbs around, the only concern is use with blood thinners such as Coumadin, since it is also a blood thinner. It is used most often for short-term memory enhancement, acting as an antioxidant, enhancing the use of oxygen and glucose—benefiting both the heart and mind. There is a specific ginkgo leaf preparation with a defined standardized biochemical profile that is suitable for this application.

Take between 40–80 mg of standardized extract in tablet or capsule form three times a day. Use only the standardized extract because current applications of ginkgo are a contemporary finding. It takes an enormous amount of plants to extract out the small amounts of flavonoids that can make a difference to brain function. Benefits increase over time. Once a "loading" dose is established for three weeks to a month, it is sometimes possible to drop down to a lesser dose that still maintains the increased mentally clarity.

The following chart shows what to look for on a label for ginkgo.

Supplement Facts

	Amount Per Day Range
Ginkgo leaf extract *(Ginkgo biloba)* standardized to 24 percent ginkgo flavonglycosides and 6 percent terpene lactones	120–180 mg
AVOID USING ANY OTHER FORM	

A summary of options for memory and concentration

In addition to the suggestions in the chart below, revisit your foundational use of vitamin E and fish oils.

memory and concentration options

OPTIONS	FORM AND DOSAGE	SIDE EFFECTS	TIME FOR EFFICACY	SERENDIPITY
Ginkgo biloba leaf extract	Standardized dose of 24 percent ginkgo flavonglycosides and 6 percent terpene lactones: 40–80 mg capsule taken up to 3x per day	When taken in higher amounts, for some, mild gastrointestinal upset, headache that goes away with use or when discontinued; blood thinner	4–6 weeks	Heart health and improved circulation for cold hands and feet (Raynaud's); relief of ringing of the ears; help for dementia

MOOD SWINGS, ANXIETY AND DEPRESSION

The years immediately preceding the last period are often the most problematic in terms of mood, anxiety and depression. Women complain they lack a "sense of well-being." Fortunately, this adjustment time tends to clear up on its own as women face both the hormonal and socio-emotional issues of this major life transition. "This too shall pass" is a byword to keep in mind. The opportunity to *renew, revamp* and *review* and the eventual stabilization of hormone levels result in older women being no more depressed than the rest of society—and often they find themselves in a better, more productive space.

perimenopause symptoms

Check symptoms or behaviors that occur throughout the month with a frequency or intensity that affects your daily activities or your ability to feel good about yourself.

- ❑ Cry a lot for no reason
- ❑ Life looks hopeless
- ❑ Miserable, sad, unhappy, blue
- ❑ Decision-making difficulties
- ❑ Anxiety
- ❑ Difficulty sleeping
- ❑ Loss of interest in things that used to bring joy
- ❑ Changes in appetite or weight
- ❑ Difficulty concentrating
- ❑ Apathetic

About St. John's wort

Side effects of St. John's wort (*Hypericum perforatum*) are far less imposing than those of antidepressant medications—which might explain its widespread use. (In 1997, $200 million worth of St. John's wort was sold in the U.S., and 111 million daily doses were sold in Germany in the same year.[10]) Extracts have been used traditionally and effectively for mild to moderate depression.[11] Research reporting it as ineffective was based on testing it for a nonrecommended purpose—*severe depression*. A number of studies support its use on moderate depression and its ability to increase brain levels of serotonin.

St. John's wort should not be combined with digoxin (a drug used for coronary problems), calcium channel blockers or lidocaine, and caution is advised with selective serotonin reuptake inhibitors (Prozac or Paxil) or monamine oxidase inhibitors. It is not a monamine oxidase inhibitor itself.[12] Photosensitivity and interaction with anesthetic agents have also been noted, and it is not to be used with birth control pills. The aerial part of the plant contains the active ingredients: hypericins, flavonoids and volatile oil.

The chart below shows what to look for on a label for St. John's wort.

Supplement Facts

	Amount Per Day

St. John's wort flowering top extract *(Hypericum perforatum)* standardized to contain 0.3 percent hypericins and 3.0 percent hyperforins **900–1,800 mg**

A summary of options for mood swings, anxiety and depression

In addition to the suggestions in the following chart, revisit your foundational use of B complex and fish oils.

mood stabilization options

OPTIONS	FORM AND DOSAGE	SIDE EFFECTS	TIME OF EFFICACY	SERENDIPITY
St. John's wort flowering tops	900–1,800 mg extract with 0.3 percent hypericins and 3 percent hyperforins	Palpitations, tremors, overly sensitive, confusion or nervousness; do not use with birth control or antiviral drugs See text above	2 week minimum	Pain relief
Progesterone cream	See end of chapter			Hot flash relief
Find support	Sharing the "journey" with friends has been shown to reduce symptoms		Generally immediately; there is always someone worse off than you!	Socialization; improves mental function and improves health generally
Exercise	Duke researchers found 30 minutes 3x per week did as well as Zoloft		Immediately	Impacts serotonin regulation and enhances chemicals that affect mood; after 6 months, 9 percent of exercisers relapsed, 30 percent pill-takers

MUSCLE AND JOINT PAIN

While muscle and joint pain is one of the most common complaints of menopause, there is little understanding to the connection with estrogen. It may be that higher hormonal doses have an immunosuppressive effect that blocks arthritic responses. More often, increased aches and pains are due to a combination of factors, which are years in the making. Poor gastrointestinal health, toxic exposure, stress, lack of exercise and poor nutrition all play their part. If you are twenty pounds overweight, you are adding one hundred pounds of pressure with each step.

aches and pains

Check symptoms or behaviors that occur throughout the month with a frequency or intensity that affects your daily activities or your ability to feel good about yourself.

- ❑ Morning stiffness
- ❑ Difficulty bending
- ❑ Joint swelling, pain, stiffness
- ❑ Joints hurt with movement
- ❑ Difficulty opening jars
- ❑ Discomfort, numbness, prickling or tingling sensations, or pain in neck, shoulder or arm

- ❑ Difficulty getting up from chair
- ❑ Difficulty reaching and holding heavy items just above head
- ❑ Increased use of painkillers

About glucosamine, chondroitin sulphate and anti-inflammatory botanicals

Glucosamine and chondroitin sulphate do not merely cover pain; they restore connective tissue. Neither are pain relievers, although they tend to alleviate pain secondarily. The best results are found when both are taken together, although chondroitin can cause nausea, indigestion or irritability in some people. Dosage is significant to the relief achieved.

Botanicals have been used for thousands of years for natural pain control. It is best to use them until pain is ameliorated and then as needed. Used continually, they have the same side-effect profile as more potent pharmaceutical pain relief drugs (NSAIDS, COX-2) and can cause gastrointestinal and kidney damage.

The chart below shows what to look for on a label for glucosamine or chondroitin sulphate.

Supplement Facts

	Amount Per Day Range
Glucosamine sulphate (as D-glucosamine sulfate KCl)	Under 120 pounds: 1,000 mg Over 120 pounds: 1,500 mg
Chondroitin sulphate	Under 120 pounds: 800 mg Over 120 pounds:1,200 mg

Sometimes trace amounts of vitamins and minerals are included. These are secondary ingredients and should not be the reason you purchase the product. Key to the success of this mixture is the regular intake of the suggested daily dosage. Be certain chondroitin sulfate is not gelatin.

The chart below shows what to look for on a label for anti-inflammatory botanicals.

Supplement Facts

	Amount Per Day Range
Turmeric rhizome extract (*Curcuma longa*) standardized to 80–95 percent curcuminoids	600–900 mg
Boswellia gum extract (*Boswellia serrata*) standardized to 70 percent boswellic acids	900–1,200 mg

Sometimes additional vitamins, minerals, antioxidants and botanicals are included. These are secondary ingredients and should not be the reason you purchase the product. Key to the success of this mixture is the regular intake of the suggested daily dosage of these specific botanicals.

A summary of options for muscle and joint pain

In addition to the suggestions in following chart, revisit your foundational use of fish oils.

aches and pains options

OPTIONS	FORM AND DOSAGE	SIDE EFFECTS	TIME FOR EFFICACY	SERENDIPITY
Glucosamine sulphate	Tablet; 1,500 mg/d; frequently pain control can be achieved at lower doses	None	Generally, within days; stimulates healthy connective tissue even if no pain relief. Use for 6 months minimum	No GI side effects like NSAIDS; glucosamine can stimulate healthy connective tissue growth whether it relieves pain or not
Chondroitin sulphate	Tablet; 1,200 mg/d	Nausea, indigestion in sensitive people	See glucosamine	Do not take with Coumadin, heparin
Boswellia/ turmeric	600–900mg/ 900–1200 mg	GI upset	Generally within days	Short term pain relief; less chance of GI upset than with pharmaceutical drugs
Massage	As scheduled			Stress relief; improves circulation of body fluids
Yoga	Class or individual practice			Stress relief; deep breathing improves total body function; stretching strengthens muscles, frees joints and muscles

LACK OF SEXUAL DESIRE: DHEA

It would be nice to be able to blame hormones for a waning sex drive or lessened pleasure. Life is never so simple, however. One's interest in sex is highly individualized and can be distanced from hormonal levels. It is always wise to look at relationship issues during any time of upheaval. Midlife women often find a renewed sense of pleasure derived from the fact they are less apt to judge themselves on their body, but to consider their entire personage in issues of self-esteem. They may also find they are able to ask for what they want, perhaps for the first time in their lives. Their male partner's less demanding sexual appetite and increasing interest in relationship tends to "level the playing field," so to speak. Couples who report the happiest marital relationships maintain a viable sex life until illness in one or both partners prevents it.

Sometimes there is no desire for sex because it is painful. Vaginal dryness is generally the concern in such cases. Solutions for this problem are discussed in this and the following chapter.

About DHEA and DHEA sulphate

DHEA is a steroid hormone that is a precursor to testosterone and estrogen. Your body normally produces 10–20 mg per day in the adrenal glands, although levels drop as we age. This is why you often see it touted as an antiaging hormone. DHEA sulphate (DHEAs) is the form that chiefly circulates in the blood stream, converting back to DHEA in the peripheral tissues. Problems with adrenal burnout, discussed in the following chapter, will naturally reduce levels of DHEA. Besides improvement of libido, there is evidence of improvement from symptoms of depression, anxiety and fatigue for some women.

Caution: Supplementation should not be considered before measuring serum or salivary levels before and then again after treatment. Since DHEA can be converted into testosterone, too high a level could result in masculinizing effects, such as a deepening voice and growth of facial hair. Such symptoms disappear when DHEA is discontinued. It is not recommended for anyone with hormone-sensitive tumors.

The following chart shows what to look for on a label for dehydroepiandosterone (DHEA).

Supplement Facts

	Amount Per Day
SPRAY Dehydroepiandosterone (DHEA)–liposome microsphere encapsulation5–25 mg	
Dehydroepiandosterone (DHEA) tablets or capsules 5–25 mg	

A summary of options for sexual desire

Along with the suggestions in the following chart, revisit your foundational use of vitamin E and fish oils.

sexual desire and function options

OPTIONS	FORM AND DOSAGE	SIDE EFFECTS	TIME FOR EFFICACY	SERENDIPITY
DHEA	Capsule: 5–25 mg/d; transmucosal spray: 5–25 mg/d; test levels before and after 6 weeks of treatment	Androgenic effects: voice deepens, excess facial hair growth; symptoms disappear when discontinued; Doses >25 mg/day, use under supervision of CAM practitioner.		Increased energy
More sex	Increased sex increases lubrication and desire			The happiest long-term relationships include a regular sexual relationship; sex is only limited by the partners' emotional and physical ability
Lubricants	Use a water soluble lubricant EVERY time you make love.			Lubricants will increase comfort (K-Y Lubricating Jelly, Astroglide or AquaLube); apply moisturizers like Replens or Gyne-Moistrin for daily comfort.
Take responsibility for making sex be what you want	May need a counselor to help you understand what you need and express it sensitively; read helpful books; short-term therapy effective (12 weeks)	Sexual counseling or couples counseling both work to improve sexuality.	Do not think it is too late or can't be changed, especially if you have never dealt with abuse issues.	A reconnection renews hope; you are empowered to know that you are responsible for insuring your pleasure.

THE SPECIAL CASE OF TRANSDERMAL NATURAL PROGESTERONE CREAM

When progesterone cream became the rage, following an article by John Lee, M.D., published in the *Lancet*,[13] I must admit I had my doubts. It was not so much what Dr. Lee said that disturbed me, but the instant hype that surrounded its use. Two premises emerged: First, that progesterone cream was the cure to just about anything a perimenopausal woman might be suffering, and second, that doctors had known this all along but were withholding it from patients for ill-gotten financial gain.

I am happy to report that although it took awhile, the definitive answer is finally in. Progesterone cream does reduce hot flashes. Some women experience an improved quality of life—getting rid of hot flashes has a tendency to do that! One study reported an improvement in or resolution of the emotional symptoms of menopause by 83 percent among those using rub-on progesterone and only 19 percent in the placebo group.[14]

No study has found an increase in bone density with transdermal progesterone, so do not plan on its use protecting you from osteoporosis or helping to prevent hyperplasia, if you are taking estrogen. Several studies verify that if kept within a level of 20–30 mg per day, progesterone is absorbed into the blood at safe levels that result in improved mood, reduced bloating and breast tenderness and help in balancing estrogen. To date there are no published studies that verify its long-term safety.[15] The FDA considers transdermal progesterone cream a *cosmetic* and advocates not exceeding 2 ounces per month and 5 mg per ounce per day; otherwise, it must be approved as a drug. Since this dosage is below a "clinically effective dose" for relief of hot flashes, it is recommended instead that you consider "natural" or "nature-identical" progesterone, prepared for relief of menopause symptoms by a compounding pharmacist, who fills an appropriate prescription at the direction of a physician.

a good for you!
Synopsis…

Should these symptom solutions not be adequate, consider the bright side: You know what *does not* work for you! Go on to chapter fifteen; it may be that other health issues, not symptoms, should be your priority. After reading to this point, you now know that "the path of least resistance" is not enough for you—at this time. Other considerations would be:

1. Did you purchase a good quality product that matched the description in the Supplement Facts box?
2. Did you adjust the dosages so they conformed with the optimal ranges?
3. Did you allow enough time to see if the product would work?
4. Did you keep up on your foundation supplement program?

15

should i go back on, get off or go on hormone replacement therapy?

OK, OK, I hear you. Your neighbor who recommended *Good for You!* as a must-read could not be happier. She has upgraded her vitamins, decided to park her car at the far end of the parking lot (to add a little exercise to her life), purchased her bottle of black cohosh—*and her hot flashes are gone!* You, on the other hand, threw out your junk food, joined the gym, have been taking your vitamins religiously, purchased your black cohosh—*and have had to start wearing a sundress in the middle of winter to keep from a total meltdown!* Besides putting up with streams of sweat, you have a vaginal infection that started right after you last made (painful) love.

I am sure there have been moments when throwing caution to the wind and restarting HRT was more than tempting. Before you do so, however, make sure you have read the instructions for your herbals and supplements carefully. Were you cautious in their selection, using the criteria of elimination outlined in chapter twelve, or is your phytoestrogen tucked into a power drink? Did you experiment a bit with dosage? Did you make your purchase at a discount store whose product was cheap, and now, looking at the label, you realize it will require taking half the bottle to reach a clinically effective dose?

Have you made any modifications in diet, exercise or to relieve stress? Or having selected carefully and made some changes, are you still miserable? If so, then there is no avoiding the big picture. Suggestions in this chapter may require a healthcare practitioner familiar with complementary or natural medicine, or a physician willing to work with you with natural and medical products and functional tests.

BUT I'M SO TIRED!

A recent study (2002) published in the journal of *The American College of Obstetricians and Gynecologists* concluded, "Symptoms typically attributed to menopause are common in elderly women [average age sixty-seven years, not over eighty]. Postmenopausal hormone therapy reduces hot flashes, trouble sleeping and vaginal dryness, but at standard doses in elderly women, is associated with vaginal discharge, genital irritation, uterine bleeding and breast symptoms." It is interesting to note that these symptoms are still considered "menopausal" and treated with hormone replacement therapy, despite the fact that most women referenced averaged eighteen years since their periods stopped. The researchers had no other explanation for such complaints or the mind-set to offer any other treatment option except HRT.[1]

I do hope that, if you have not already done an evaluation of your baseline health issues, you will do so soon. As we have pointed out, there are many things that "look" like menopause—"menopause mimics," so to speak. They so closely resemble menopause symptomology that it takes a discerning eye—often a professional one—to make the distinction. What we saw most frequently in our clinic were problems with thyroid function. Is it possible your lack of success with natural products for menopausal symptomology is related to thyroid problems?

a checklist for thyroid function

- ❑ Hot/cold flashes
- ❑ Cold
- ❑ Forgetfulness
- ❑ Insomnia
- ❑ Overwhelming tiredness
- ❑ Agitation
- ❑ Depression
- ❑ Aches and pains
- ❑ Upper eyelids look swollen/quickly
- ❑ Muscles are weak, cramp and/or tremble
- ❑ Feel that heart beats slowly
- ❑ Dryness, discoloration of skin and/or hair

- ❑ Voice seems to be deepening
- ❑ Outer third lid of eyebrow is thinning or disappearing
- ❑ Swelling in the neck area
- ❑ Reaction time seems slowed down
- ❑ Low sexual desire
- ❑ Slow-moving and sluggish
- ❑ Constipation
- ❑ Thick, brittle nails
- ❑ Weight gain for no apparent reason
- ❑ Premenstrual tension

Diagnosis of thyroid issues requires laboratory tests, family history and consideration of symptoms. Problems with the thyroid gland increase considerably past one's fortieth birthday and may result in an underactive (hypothyroid) or overactive (hyperthyroid) condition. The most common form, hypothyroidism, is easily rectified by medication within one to three months. If not, you could have a problem converting your thyroid (T-4 to T-3) from one form to another, requiring two different thyroid medications.

A MIMIC FOR MOST OF US—ADRENOPAUSE

Especially with Type A, highly stressed women (remember Diane in chapter eleven), or those who have lived with much stress or illness, "midlife angst" not readily taken care of by the usual menopause interventions can often be attributed to adrenal problems. The causes are multiple and usually have been years in the making. HRT was decidedly unhelpful for such women. The Adrenocortex Stress Profile provides measurements of imbalance in cortisol and DHEA, their bioavailability and a means to measure the effectiveness of therapy. (See chapter eight.)

A genuine effort to live a calmer life is essential for medicinal therapy to work. Restoring adrenal function and rebalancing cortisol may take weeks to months. It took years to compromise adrenal function, and patience is required to undo the damage. Interventions for addressing unhealthy adrenal patterns are almost completely dependent on functional or complementary medicine concepts.

---

symptoms of adrenopause

- ❏ Lingering fatigue after exertion or stress
- ❏ Easily fatigued
- ❏ Sleep problems
- ❏ Craving for salty foods
- ❏ Sensitive to minor changes in weather and surroundings
- ❏ Dizzy when rising or standing up
- ❏ Dark eye circles

IT ISN'T JUST A STOMACHACHE

Years of dealing with toxic chemicals, a high-fat, low-fiber diet, allergens, illnesses and medications (NSAIDs, corticosteroids) break down digestive health. But damage can occur quickly as a result of certain medications (antacids, gastric acid inhibitors) and antibiotic use. An antibiotic cannot tell the difference between the estimated five hundred types of helpful and harmful bacteria normally residing in the intestinal tract. It can disrupt the healthy balance (a condition known as *dysbiosis*) of resident bacteria to the point that the ability of the gastrointestinal lining to serve its protective and immune functions is compromised. Most noticeably, there are digestive upset, gas, bloating, yeast and bladder infections, and perhaps irritable bowel syndrome (IBS). Depending on the mix of medications over your lifetime, symptoms seemingly unrelated to your GI tract, like connective tissue and joint problems or decline in mental functioning, can result. Since by now you have a concept of functional medicine and view the body function as an interactive web, it is understandable that a disrupted bowel can both prevent interventions from working and trigger symptoms.

dysbiosis/leaky gut

❑ Indigestion
❑ Burpy
❑ Bloating following meals
❑ Discomfort, pain or cramps in lower abdominal area
❑ Generally constipated
❑ Alternate between constipation and diarrhea
❑ Stool is hard, dry; no urge for bowel movement
❑ Almost continual need to have a bowel movement
❑ Digestive problems subside with rest and relaxation

A "damaged" intestinal tract, sometimes referred to as a "leaky gut," can contribute to the "simmer" effect or low-grade inflammation, impairing the proper absorption of food, supplements and medication. Many of your aches and pains, particularly arthritis pain, are made worse by it.

There are products on the market that can help you heal a damaged gastrointestinal tract. They are called "probiotics." They consist of live bacteria in the form of powder or tablets and are present in small amounts in foods such as yogurt and milk.[2] The two most beneficial probiotics, also called "friendly flora" or "friendly bacteria," are *Lactobacillus acidophilus* and *bifidobacteria*.[3] Realizing health benefits from probiotic supplementation require that you take billions (10–120 billion) of live viable bacteria per day. Products vary greatly in quality. If you want to explore using probiotics, use the following checklist:

choosing quality probiotics

- Use good science—demonstration of human health benefits for the bacteria in the product through published research
- Adequate potency—minimum of ten billion live *Lactobacillus acidophilus* and *bifidobacteria* per serving
- Viability—proof that when taken orally the bacteria survive transit through the stomach and small intestines
- Third-party laboratory assays verifying the live cell count and bacteria viability
- Refrigeration during the shipping and storage of the product to ensure the third-party assays

There is a secondary but connected problem if the intestinal tract does not do its work—the liver is overrun in its efforts to *detoxify* and render harmless countless microbial, hormonal or chemical molecules. *Bifidobacteria* have been shown to enhance immune systems even among the elderly.[4] We have seen the scary possibilities when inadequate bowel bacteria or liver function results in estrogen being broken down to unfavorable metabolites. You owe it to yourself to do the little it takes to ensure bowel health.

At our clinic, the addition of probiotics proved miraculous for many women—even for those who were reluctant to make other lifestyle changes. We used the highly researched NCFM strain of *Lactobacillus acidophilus* in combination with a specific strain of *Bifidobacteria lactis*. There were some women, however, who required medicinal detoxification—women who had undergone chemotherapy, suffered longstanding chronic diseases or who were highly allergenic. (Note: If you desire help and medical food products to improve gut function, we recommend an FDA-approved program from Metagenics, 100 Avenida La Pata, San Clemente, CA 92673, toll free: 800-692-9400 or www.metagenics.com.)

THE SUGAR CONNECTION

Another possibility for experiencing failure of "menopause" treatments is insulin resistance. When an excess of processed, high-glycemic foods are overeaten or not balanced nutritionally, the system is overwhelmed by excessive blood sugar. The pancreas responds with excess insulin, and the cells become "insulin resistant." Faulty blood sugar metabolism impacts your weight, shape (body composition or muscle to fat ratio), energy levels, blood pressure, cholesterol and cardiovascular health—and, according to a very new study, your memory.[5] Blood sugar levels are controlled by eating small, low-glycemic meals, exercising and maintaining a healthy weight.

blood sugar imbalance

When you miss meals or go without food for an extended period of time, do you experience any of the following symptoms?

- ❑ Sense of weakness
- ❑ Anxiety when you get hungry
- ❑ Tingling sensation in your hands
- ❑ A sensation of your heart beating too quickly or forcefully
- ❑ Shaky, jittery, hands trembling
- ❑ Wake up at night feeling restless
- ❑ Agitation, easily upset, nervous
- ❑ Poor memory, forgetful
- ❑ Confused or disoriented

- ❑ Dizzy, faint
- ❑ Cold or numb
- ❑ Mild headaches or head pounding
- ❑ Blurred vision or double vision
- ❑ Feel clumsy and uncoordinated
- ❑ Sudden profuse sweating and/or your skin feels clammy
- ❑ Nightmares possibly related to going to bed on an empty stomach

ARE HORMONES THE CHOICE?

So, here you are; you admit that it is probable that one or more of these health issues are at work, which could possibly explain why you do not feel well and why the usual menopause interventions are not relieving symptoms. Natural solutions sound good but seem like a lot of work. Maybe there is a part of you that is still more interested in the path of least resistance than getting to the core of what is really going on. Could it be that after reading all these chapters and learning what functional medicine is, the desire for a silver bullet is still strong? Like the siren in *Ulysses*, does the call of a quick fix remain mesmerizing and compelling? If that is so, let's review what we "finally" know as of 2003 about hormone replacement therapy.

Dismal results of HRT study

As previously noted, in July 2002, *The Journal of the American Medical Association* (*JAMA*) reported that the Women's Health Initiative (WHI), a study of 161,809 postmenopausal women (fifty to seventy-nine years old) was canceled—at least a portion of it. The women had been placed on estrogen/progestin, or estrogen only, and monitored for coronary heart disease, venous thrombotic events, breast cancer, colon cancer and fractures. When a predetermined "global index" that measures when risk outweighs benefit reached the critical point, the estrogen/progestin arm of the study was discontinued.

The alarming WHI results do not apply to every conceivable combination and type of hormone replacement. The outcome pertains to the estrogen *Premarin* and the progestin *Provera*. But realistically, other choices, nature-identical or synthetic, cannot be proven to be better and safer, at least at this time.

Consider *this...* Long-term combined HRT (five years) appears to increase fibroids in women with a BMI under 24 (thin women).[6]

The WHI can be considered a true "prevention" study because the women involved had few of the illnesses for which they were being tested. This monumental trial is an example of "evidence-based research" replacing conventional wisdom. It has been observed that "the reaction to any new scientific finding is proportional to the strength of the accepted dogma that it overturns."[7] While the results of the study have been dismissed as dealing with "older" women (the average age was sixty-three), risks were elevated in *all* ages of women. While absolute risk for any one woman is small, when extrapolated to millions, the numbers become substantial, especially with length of use. The areas of benefit (colorectal cancer and hip fracture) do not statistically offset the disadvantages. This is especially true because there are other options—safe lifestyle interventions with no downside, which help in the prevention and treatment of these conditions.

Despite the naysayers, there is no getting around the reality that the WHI was a well-designed study. The National Institutes of Health (NIH) set it up with several research arms. The estrogen-only portion of the study is still underway because it has not reached a point where risks outweigh benefits. It is a smaller trial, and it may be that risk milestones have not been reached or that it is indeed the combination of estrogen with a progestin that is the culprit behind the danger.

However, such a conclusion might be premature because the recently published "Million Women Study" found women ages fifty to sixty-four who took HRT had an increase in breast cancer whether they had taken estrogen alone and regardless of the type or method of delivery.[8]

The belief that HRT might not have all the protective benefits it was touted to have began to crumble with the HERS trials. But since the publication of the WHI study, two other smaller analyses have conveyed the same dismal results for heart protection. One study demonstrated even worse clinical outcomes and more rapid disease progression.[9] When considering this preponderance of evidence, it is clear that women who are on HRT to prevent heart disease should stop. Those solely on HRT for osteoporosis risk or disease should, with their physicians, consider discontinuing its use. Young women with premature menopause and/or those with hysterectomy are advised to continue its use. They, along with older women who are on estrogen only, should keep close track of the outcome of the WHI estrogen-only trial due to end in 2005. Since the NIH is still analyzing data, and recommendations may change, it is wise to keep in touch with your doctor and to check the NIH Web site periodically.

onsider *this...* A recent study showed that flaxseed was as effective as HRT in improving mild menopause symptoms.[10]

TEN BIG HRT QUESTIONS WOMEN ARE ASKING

If you have questions concerning HRT, consider the discussion below in answer to ten of the most common questions women are asking.

1. How do I go off hormone replacement?

There is no reason you cannot simply stop taking hormones. You will not suffer any untoward medical consequence. In fact, there are many women who cannot tell the difference from one day to the next. That said, other women will undoubtedly suffer through some uncomfortable symptoms—that prove bearable—and the deed is done. For those whose symptomology measures on the Richter scale, it is wise to abandon the "grin-and-bear-it" approach and go back on hormones and taper off gradually. It is probably wiser (and from a natural medicine perspective, easier on your body) to taper off. If you are on the highest dose of estrogen (0.625 mg), you could cut your pills in two or ask your physician for a prescription for a lower dose (0.3 mg). Should you be fearful of symptoms being more than you can bear, try alternating days (0.625 with 0.3 mg) for a month, working toward the lower dose only and tapering off from there. The same "tapering" can be used with the "patch." Most women simply extend their time between pills until they feel comfortable enough to stop completely.

2. Is there a safe length of time for taking HRT?

The general consensus is that should you decide to use HRT for symptom relief (hot flashes and vaginal dryness only), or you are already taking it, it ought to be continued for the shortest time possible. Sophisticated diagnostic tests may eventually delineate risk of HRT for every individual. Since risk increases with each additional year of use, an effort to taper off every six months is advised. Basically, with a few individual exceptions, no responsible medical practitioner (or their professional organization) is recommending hormone use for longer than three to five years, with four years being more of a consensus.

A caution is in order, however, that while breast cancer risk is not *diagnosed* until the fifth year of HRT use, there is no proof it has not been set in motion earlier. You should also be aware that the greatest risk for cardiovascular events occurs within the first year. As yet we do not know if this negative effect is ameliorated by using a nature-identical (micronized) progesterone versus Provera to balance the estrogen. This will be determined in the future.

3. If I decide to take HRT longer than four years, or if I have already been on HRT for more than four years, what health risks or benefits do I face?

Consider the results in the following chart and discussion of HRT use to determine what health risks/benefits you may expect.

Women's Health Initiative Study Outcomes

OUTCOMES	HAZARD RATIO	INCREASED RISK IN 10,000 WOMEN TAKING PREMPRO FOR ONE YEAR
Coronary heart disease (CHD)	+29 percent	7 more CHD events
Stroke	+41 percent	8 more strokes
Venous thromboembolism/ blood clots (VTE)	+111 percent	18 more VTEs
Breast cancer	+26 percent	8 more invasive breast cancers
Colorectal cancer	-37 percent	6 fewer colorectal cancers
Hip fracture	-37 percent	5 fewer hip fractures

Adapted from "Writing Group for the Women's Health Initiative Investigation," *JAMA* 288 (2002): 321.

A large Swedish study begun in 1990 and completed in 2003 (thirty thousand women, one of every eight Swedish women aged twenty-five through sixty-five with 227,000 person-years of follow-up) confirmed the WHI study conclusion that HRT increases breast cancer. After four years of estrogen/progestin use, the risk was equivalent to half that associated with carrying the BRAC1 gene. With forty-eight months use, there was an 80 percent greater risk than never-users for breast cancer. Risk with combined use was lower than that of sequential use; progestin-only use also increased cancer, but estrogen-only did not.[11]

Besides the increase in breast cancer, stroke and blood clots, it should be noted that women in the WHI had an 80 percent higher rate of cardiovascular incidents than the placebo group the first year, which declined to 15 percent the second year. This mirrored the HERs II trial results. It is theorized that the increase in heart problems could not be due to atherosclerosis because of the short period of time; therefore, it is likely explained by inflammation or interaction with homocysteine factors. Transdermal (the patch) estrogen-progestin therapy increases rates of cardiovascular events in women with heart disease just like the pill.[12] Hormone replacement increases dry eye with a significantly higher risk with each three years of use.[13] After twenty years on HRT, the relative risk of ovarian cancer is 3.2 where 1 is no risk. This translates into a 220 percent increase.[14]

In May 2003, another arm of the Women's Health Initiative was halted (Women's Health Initiative Memory Study: A Randomized Controlled Trial [WHIM]), when it was found that the hormone combination doubled the risk for dementia in women age sixty-five or older and did not prevent mild cognitive impairment. Translated to a population of ten thousand women taking the combined therapy, that would mean an additional twenty-three cases of dementia per year.[15]

4. I have done as much as I am willing to do, including natural interventions, but hot flashes are leaving me drenched with sweat, with my heart racing, and an inability to sleep. I am going to go back on HRT. Can I reduce the risk?

Again, what you can count on hormones doing is relieving (by about 80 percent) hot flashes and vaginal/urinary distress.[16] There is ongoing research to determine if there are subgroups of women who can safely derive benefit from HRT. Obviously, from the above results, if you have cardiovascular issues or a family history of breast cancer, HRT is not an option for you.

If you do not have those risk factors, one consideration that relates to safe use is your age. If you are younger (and likely more symptomatic), you may have less risk. A woman of fifty is 50 percent less likely to have a disease influenced by hormones than a sixty-year-old woman. The following chart demonstrates this, using WHI results:

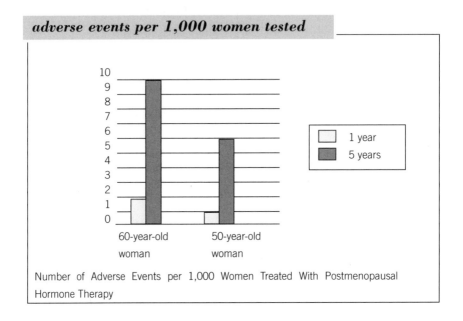

adverse events per 1,000 women tested

1 year
5 years

60-year-old woman
50-year-old woman

Number of Adverse Events per 1,000 Women Treated With Postmenopausal Hormone Therapy

Clearly, age is a factor in risk with hormone use. If you have not first tried controlling hot flashes and vaginal distress naturally, you should do so before starting HRT. Once they begin, hot flashes last about one or two years in most women.[17] Therefore, it may be possible from an age perspective for the majority who are unable to relieve symptoms naturally to use HRT for a very short period of time to manage hot flashes when they are at their worst. Know that since they do not last forever, you should try to wean yourself off HRT as soon as possible.

Should you decide to use HRT, select the lowest effective dose. You might consider transdermal (the patch) estrogen to reduce bad-girl metabolites. Persons with gallstones or a poorly functioning liver or digestive tract should certainly give this consideration. Make sure your estrogen is soy-based. Equine (Premarin) and human estrogens are quite different. Also, pay attention to the progestogen you take; both animal and human trials have shown increased safety and effectiveness of micronized progesterone (nature-identical) when compared to progestin (Provera).

If you are a woman with dense breast tissue, think twice about HRT for hot flash relief. Dense breast tissue is a sign of active estrogen activity and of extra breast estrogen and should make you hesitant to add still more estrogen. Dense breast tissue is a breast cancer risk factor that is actually higher than the risk from HRT. Also, consider passing on using HRT if you are overweight, because you make extra estrogen already.

5. How do I cope with vaginal dryness and urinary incontinence?

Vaginal dryness and problems with urinary control are indications of estrogen deprivation. The vulva, vagina, urethra, bladder neck and bladder are rich in estrogen receptors and responsive to local hormonal therapy. The problem is progressive, and when treatment is stopped, it is almost always likely to return. This means that if you happen to be a woman who has been unable to resolve what is known medically as "urogenital atrophy" with the suggestions mentioned in the chapters on natural solutions, you may find that regular application of a hormone directly into the vagina is essential.

I am one of those women. Discontinuation of hormone therapy resulted in spastic urinary pain that felt as if I had a serious urinary or bladder infection, although I did not. Bleeding following intercourse or pain as a result of coitus are also common as a result of loss of collagen, fat and the vagina's inability to retain water. Changes in pH open the way for increased infection, itching and irritation. After an initial "loading" dose, creams or tablets used one to three times a week are enough to maintain vaginal health, which is achieved usually within a month or in severe cases within six months.

Because the dosage is low and little hormone is absorbed into the bloodstream, estrogen can be given without progesterone even in a woman with an intact uterus.[18] Maintaining the thickness of the vaginal walls contributes to keeping the hormones localized—a good reason for not letting urogenital atrophy get out of hand. Nonhormonal moisturizers and water-soluble lubricants decrease pain and irritation but do not fix the underlying cause.

Your physician can give you a prescription for vaginal estrogen tablets (Vagifem), or you can use a three-month estrogen-releasing ring (Estring— recommended for two years) or creams (Estrace, Dienestrol or other soy-based cream).[19] To further allay your fears of this limited use of hormones, a compounding pharmacist can make creams in a nonallergenic base that contain "natural" estrogen, progesterone or even testosterone. There is a new vaginal ring (Femring) that relieves vaginal dryness and hot flashes and acts systemically; it requires a progestogen balance and generally acts like a low-dose oral HRT.[20] Do not be embarrassed to bring this problem to the attention of your physician. Do note, however, that urinary incontinence can have other causes such as weight, number of children, diabetes or smoking.

6. Should I consider a SERM?

We have spoken of phytoestrogens in soy and other plant sources acting like SERMs (selective estrogen receptor modulators). Here we are referring to the use of pharmaceutically derived substitutes for estrogen developed for specific purposes. At the moment, two are used extensively—Tamoxifen and Raloxifene. Neither are estrogens; they work selectively on estrogen receptors. Tamoxifen is an antiestrogen used to prevent or treat breast cancer for up to five years.

Besides its beneficial effect on breast cancer, the toxic effects to consider include increased risk of endometrial cancer, problems with clotting (thromboembolic events) and increased hot flashes in some women. New research indicates smaller doses reduce negative side effects. If you are a high-risk woman, you may be asked to participate in Tamoxifen prevention studies.

Raloxifene produces favorable responses in bone and lipids, while lowering the incidence of breast cancer—sounds ideal. However, the MORE study (Multiple Outcomes of Raloxifene Evaluation) reported that it did not reduce fractures other than the spine; it tripled the risk of venous thrombotic disease (blood clot and stroke) and did not help cognition while increasing the incidence of hot flashes and leg cramps.[21] A recent study with Raloxifene showed it negatively affects risk factors associated with cholesterol.[22] Both of these pharmaceutical SERMs are known to increase hot flashes and vaginal dryness. The silver bullet has yet to be found. At present, there is no long-term evidence that they are safer than HRT, and ACOG recommends their use strictly for their FDA-approved use. (Note: Before you begin treatment with a SERM, review what is known so far at Medscape Women's Health eJournal 7(5), 2002: www.medscape.com/viewarticle/441559.)

7. Do "nature-identical" hormones put me at the same risk as traditional pharmaceutical versions?

Quite honestly, this question cannot be answered. Other than the greater lipid-protective benefits, ability to reduce hot flashes and its lower side-effect profile, micronized (nature-identical) progesterone is about the only "natural" hormone with some support in the scientific literature. Most estrogen products, whether from a large pharmaceutical house or a compounding pharmacy, are soy-based. Many in the alternative community feel that using the weakest form of estrogen, estriol, is a better choice. When estriol is given as continuous application and at effective dosage, the concentration is equal to that of estradiol and therefore can produce the same biologic responses.[23] Lyra and I continue to stress the importance of not seeking a "new" estrogen but using lifestyle, therapeutic nutrition and botanicals as your safest choices.

8. I want to take HRT because it will improve (or has improved) my sense of well-being. Is this not a sound reason?

The Women's Health Initiative's comprehensive study of quality of life issues and menopause took into account physical function, inability to participate in usual activities, bodily pain, energy and fatigue, emotional or mental problems, health and social functioning. Additionally, they studied depression, sleep, sexual and cognitive function and symptoms associated with menopause, such as hot flashes. The study group was comprised of a large randomized trial of ethnically and geographically diverse post-menopausal women. And do you know what they found? "Estrogen plus progestin had no clinically meaningful benefits on health-related quality of life or other psychosocial outcomes."[24] A small, but statistically significant, benefit was seen after one year with improvement of sleep, physical functioning and bodily pain, but did not reach criteria for clinical effectiveness; those differences were only 1–4 percent over baseline scores. In other words, other interventions worked better or as well.

If there is no benefit, the risk you take cannot be justified. The modest sleep benefit and hot flash relief did not improve other aspects of quality of life. Other studies have demonstrated that quality-of-life issues are improved by many nonhormone interventions, including education about menopause and losing weight, which reduces risk and aches and pains.[25] When an arm of the HERS trial tested quality of life, they discovered that women who took HRT had lowered physical function and a trend toward increased fatigue. The only women who weren't shown to be worse off were those who began the study with hot flashes and sleep issues and found some relief.[26] Cumulatively, these studies demonstrate that you are unlikely to "feel better" on HRT, and as many women have long attested, may feel worse.

9. Are birth control pills a problem?

The Women's Care Study found that oral contraceptives do not increase breast cancer risk regardless of duration, age, dosage or family history.[27] They do increase the risk for thrombosis, and if you smoke, the risk for stroke, systemic lupus erythematosus and cardiovascular events like hypertension is also increased. Some physicians have begun prescribing low-dose birth control pills to manage perimenopausal symptoms. Birth control pills contain far less hormone than HRT. One of the major benefits is the reduction in ovarian cancer, particularly with higher progestin dosage.[28]

10. Can I safely take a progestogen and discontinue my estrogen?

Progestogen is only given to help prevent overgrowth of the lining of the uterus when taking estrogen. Other than its transdermal use for hot flash prevention, there is no reason you need to take it. Estrogen stimulates ductal growth, and progestogen is necessary for breast lobule formation. It increases breast density.[29] Whether or not the type of progestogen makes a difference has not been determined. So far the negative outcomes are associated with progestins. The Postmenopausal Estrogen/Progestin Interventions (PEPI) trials which, like the WHI, studied average to low-risk women, demonstrated that the metabolic effects of estrogen were not significantly affected by micronized progesterone, but were by progestin (MPA).[30] Incidentally, testosterone levels in the blood have been found to be associated with postmenopausal breast cancer.[31]

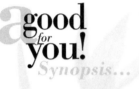

1. Are you clear about the criteria for hormone replacement use?

2. Does your health history preclude hormone use?

3. Have you been able to let go of what HRT promised and accept the reality of what it does?

4. If your doctor insists it is fine for you to remain on HRT, what do you think?

PART IV
The Long-Term Perspective

While symptom relief is lovely, looking after your health does not end there. As you age, your body is susceptible to diseases that, while not limited to an older crowd, tend to appear more frequently—heart disease, complications of obesity such as metabolic syndrome (Syndrome X), osteoporosis, Alzheimer's and even breast cancer.

Understanding the role of inflammation in such illnesses and how therapeutic lifestyle interventions can profoundly affect their onset and severity is essential to wellness.

Chapter sixteen evaluates preventative strategies for fighting the big risks.

Chapter seventeen concludes with some thoughts on aging and how your spiritual viewpoint fits into a healthy lifestyle.

The epilogue contains a perspective on potential new "silver bullets."

16

fighting the big risks without hormones

The focus of *Good for You!* has not been on maintaining perpetual youth; our focus is on aging with grace and optimal well-being. While we make suggestions, there is no set magic formula or special product to buy. Your results only minimally depend on the latest and greatest from the biggest medical research center. Many health answers lie simply in what your grandmother or mother tried to tell you: eat vegetables, and exercise. To a great extent, what you decide to do about your health will determine the quality of a full one-third of your life—your "third age."

One of the realities of becoming a "third-ager" is the possible diagnosis of chronic diseases. Osteoporosis, cancer, heart disease, arthritis, inflammatory bowel problems, metabolic syndrome and Alzheimer's disease are markers of a body that has done a lot of living. The cards dealt—our genes—once considered to predict our destiny, are no longer believed to be the masters of our fate. More importantly, it has been concluded, is our gene expression, the message genes send as a result of lifestyle.

And as we have been stating throughout this book, the message many a gene is able to send is modified by lifestyle. Your attitude about life, your spirituality, what you order from the thousands of menu options or choose from the grocery shelf, whether or not you walk your dog or send it out the doggy door, all have the power to modify gene expression. Whether you fret over "spilt milk" or simply clean up the mess, and whether you live near a toxic dumpsite, eat organically or bathe your lungs in polluted air from your cigarettes, all have much to do with how your third age unfolds.

Bodies, after years of battling internal and external toxins and plain old wear and tear, begin to break down. Nothing has been designed to last for-ever, and our earthly bodies are no exception. The pressure to avoid aging and diseases associated with aging drove much of the HRT mania. The option is not either to deny age or head for the nearest wheelchair; our best choice is to take stock and become the healthiest "old you" you can be.

THE KEYS TO "FIRE FIGHTING"

Scientists are increasingly acknowledging something that is very basic to a functional medicine or a traditional Chinese medicine (TCM) practi-tioner's viewpoint—body chemistry and function are a maze of interacting events that take action both to prevent and cause illness. A disease or poor function in one system is inevitably going to affect and perhaps undermine other aspects of one's health, or our interventions can undermine our health, as we saw with HRT. The incredible balance of body chemistry, designed for our good, can be nudged to an imbalance, resulting in harm.

Friendly fire

Here is one example of how that imbalance works in your body. Think back to a time when you were out to dinner and food lodged between your teeth. Not wanting to pick your teeth in front of your son's future in-laws, you did some ballet moves with your tongue to dislodge most of whatever was there. You go home and give your teeth their nightly two-minute scrub, but are too tired to floss. A tiny speck escapes your probing, and by morning an area of your gum is reddened, swollen and sore.

While you overlooked this minute invader, your body did not. It sends out an arsenal of macrophages (your body's killer cells) and T cells (white blood cells) to annihilate the attacker with a killer dose of chemicals that also set in motion other lifesaving mechanisms. You floss and rinse, and within a day the pain and redness subside. This protective, albeit inflamed, response has been dubbed "friendly fire." Your immune system detected a danger and swiftly responded to minimize damage. It did what it was designed to do.

Out-of-control fire

But as you well know, fire, when not contained, becomes very unfriendly. Inflammatory "fire," when out of control in the body, becomes a major factor in the majority of diseases we encounter as we age. So what is the consequence of deciding not to floss your teeth? You may not develop a sore gum that indicates an invasion of nasty bacteria, but that does not mean you do not have a "mini-war" going on. Instead of your inflammatory process shutting down and resting until the next true assault, it remains hyped-up, but below your awareness, and prepared to act, though it is not clear why. And act it does. With no invasion to attend to, it begins to attack healthy tissue.

The healthy tissue this harmful inflammation goes after could be within the vessels of the heart. How does this happen? The low-grade infection in your mouth (or infection from some other source) can send out orders to produce more troops (macrophages and T cells), which proceed to attack LDL in your bloodstream, causing it to produce fatty, frothy plaque that digs into artery walls. It stays there, perhaps for years, until immune chemicals, working inside the plaque, literally pop the seal and release blood-clot-producing factors that glom to material in the blood. These factors quickly form clots that sail along until they get stuck in arteries in the neck or brain, causing a stroke, or they block an artery in the heart, resulting in a heart attack. In fact, inflammation is now thought to be the major cause of plaque rupture.

While atherosclerosis is the main cause of plaque development, half of all heart attacks occur in people whose cholesterol levels put them in the safe "atta-girl" category, two-thirds of which have no major artery blockage. These attacks are caused by overzealous inflammatory processes, so essential for our protection, which become an uncontrolled fire with catastrophic results.

Inflammation in disease

It is understood that inflammation processes are at work with cancer. Lengthy exposure to internal or external toxins or too much sun, among other known cancer-causing agents, appear to switch on the immune system, wherein inflammatory processes, ironically, end up feeding and protecting the rebel cancer cells. Long-term damage from inflammation due to severe heartburn or inflammatory bowel disease increases cancer risk.

Arthritis is a known inflammatory disease. It was the discovery that arthritis patients who fought their inflamed joints with anti-inflammatory medication like NSAIDs and aspirin had lowered incidence of Alzheimer's that first tipped scientists to its inflammation connection, as well. Even diabetes is suspect because especially potent proteins involved in inflammation interfere with insulin's ability to regulate blood sugar properly. It is speculated that inflammation may even cause the liver to produce too much blood sugar.

Reducing inflammation

Obviously, as we get older, reduction of inflammation is essential to insure optimal health. The really good news is that you already know what you must do. Good nutrition and selective supplementation provide the foundation. There is no getting around the fact that to maintain inflammatory processes as no more than "friendly fire" requires that you avoid fast food. Eating a high-fat/high-carbohydrate meal will elevate inflammatory processes as long as four hours after your meal. If you stopped at MacDonald's for lunch and then at four o'clock had a muffin or doughnut with your friend at the coffee shop, it is possible for inflammatory processes to be elevated for another three or four hours, meaning seven to eight hours of increased chance for damage. The healthier you are, the less damage such a trip to the "wild side" will do. But if you are at risk for heart disease, are diabetic or arthritic, such indulgence could be very risky.

It is interesting to note that exercise actually triggers an increased inflammatory response. But your body, recognizing a good thing when it sees it, immediately sets in motion the production of antioxidants that ultimately reduce the inflammatory response to "friendly fire" levels. Because inflammation involves changes in gastrointestinal function, liver detoxification and the immune, nervous and endocrine system function, anything that improves overall health, such as exercise, will improve inflammatory processes.

You may have noted a connection between what you eat and increased joint pain. This is because the gastrointestinal tract plays an important role in both local and systemic inflammation. Imbalance of gut bacteria can lead to inflammation throughout your body. Inflammation is lowered when attention is paid to lifestyle, environment, diet and stress management. Study the chart below to determine how to decrease harmful inflammation processes.

keeping the fire friendly

THINGS THAT INCREASE INFLAMMATION	THINGS THAT DECREASE INFLAMMATION
The wrong fat: omega-6 in corn, safflower, sunflower and sesame oils	Good fat: omega-3 in olive and canola oils; salmon, walnuts and flaxseed; raw material for making anti-inflammatory hormones
Fast food; high-fat, low-fiber, processed, contaminated food	Probiotics restore intestinal bacteria balance.
Your own fat cells produce chemicals that direct inflammation processes.	Healthy fat/lean ratio; exercise produces antioxidants, lowers C-reactive protein.
Normal LDL plus inflammatory risk factors and high LDL trigger immune system reactions leading to heart attack, stroke and high blood pressure.	Nitric oxide maintains health of vessel lining, preventing plague formation; exercise, Mediterranean-style diet, statins, ACE inhibitors, beta-blockers, aspirin, lowering blood pressure

THINGS THAT INCREASE INFLAMMATION	THINGS THAT DECREASE INFLAMMATION
Low-grade infections like gum disease, bronchitis, cold sores or ulcer-producing bacteria	Soy, exercise, echinacea, adequate rest, reduction of stress, vitamin C to increase immunity
Stress hormones like cortisol and adrenaline keep immune and inflammatory processes from turning off.	Meditation, prayer, yoga and massage reduce stress hormones.
Lack of vegetables and fruits	Fruits and vegetables contain phytonutrients, especially antioxidants and flavonoids that block inflammation-promoting hormones, and some (raspberries, raisins, prunes, broccoli, zucchini, green peppers, tomato sauce) may even reduce pain naturally or calm inflammation; bright colors and berries are winners; spices such as turmeric contain the anti-inflammatory curcumin.
Too many high-glycemic foods, processed foods or fast foods	Whole grains, oatmeal, foods that improve glucose levels
Very high-protein diets	Soy protein; genistein/daidzen have anti-inflammatory properties and lower free radicals that cause microscopic damage and inflammation.
Sugary soft drinks	Green or black tea, orange or cranberry juice, red wine
HRT[1]	Black cohosh (mild anti-inflammatory)
Cortisol and NSAID use with gastrointestinal upset	Glucosamine sulfate and chondroitin sulfate, Co-Q_{10}; botanicals: oleanolic acid to reduce swelling, rosemary extract *(Rosmarinus officinalis)*, turmeric *(Curcuma longa)*, boswellia *(Boswellia serrata)* and ginger *(Zingiber officinale)*
Vitamin depletion	Vitamins E, K and A; carotene, zinc, selenium

How on fire are you?

There are basically three stages to inflammation. The first may be considered the *simmering* stage, characterized by mild, intermittent discomfort, which is amplified by trips to fast-food places. The second stage is when the flames are fanned and aches, pains and headaches become a big part of your life. In the third stage, flames are raging when a high-sensitivity C-reactive protein test (hs-CRP) can measure the body's inflammation. Such a test is a marker for all-cause mortality.

Evidence from the Women's Health Initiative has shown the hs-CRP test accurately predicts impending heart attack and stroke more precisely than elevated low-density lipoprotein.[2] This does not mean that LDL is insignificant, just that it measures different risk. Both tests are recommended. It also appears that C-reactive protein actually participates in arterial disease, and those who register high levels will have it in their plaques.

---

onsider *this...* Obese women who lost weight also reduced vascular inflammatory markers.[3]

When the body attacks itself

Essentially when inflammatory (or other) processes go bad and disrupt function by attacking healthy cells, the person is said to have an autoimmune disease. In such cases, T cells fail to make the distinction of "you" and "not you." Women are ten times more likely than men to be afflicted. Seventy-five percent of rheumatoid arthritis sufferers are women, as are 70–80 percent of people with lupus and up to 90 percent with multiple sclerosis. Other autoimmune disorders include Hashimoto's thyroiditis, eczema and psoriasis.[4]

With arthritis, which is the leading cause of disability among adults in the United States, the misguided immune system targets the joints.[5] Pain is controlled in most cases by anti-inflammatory medications and, in severe cases, prednisone or cyclosporine to "turn down" the activity of the immune system. Because these drugs have high side-effect profiles, we recommend that you cut down or eliminate their use with natural options.

As you might expect from the preponderance of women sufferers, hormones have a role. Studies of HRT (estrogen alone or in combination with progesterone) and quality-of-life measures report that HRT aggravates osteoarthritis.[6] In the fourth century B.C., Hippocrates used willow bark and other plants to produce the first nonsteroidal anti-inflammatory (NSAIDs). As we have noted previously, these drugs work, but at a price. The biggest danger of NSAIDs is gastrointestinal bleeding. The second harmful effect is kidney stress; the most widespread is an upset gastrointestinal tract. Consider natural interventions, exercise and stress relief first.

SELF-DEFENSE FOR SERIOUS RISKS

The following discussions briefly describe the levels of risk for life-threatening disease and offer effective ways to lower the risk and, in some cases, eliminate it.

Keeping the heart healthy

1. The risk

The *2002 Heart and Stroke Statistical Update* (American Heart Association) reported that over 60 million Americans have some form of cardiovascular disease—450,000 women died with it in 1999. While women are slower (by about ten years) to develop heart disease, it is a woman's leading cause of death. In fact, since 1984, more women die of heart attacks annually than men. Sixty-three percent of women who die suddenly had no prior symptoms.[7] A woman is ten times more likely to die from heart disease than breast cancer. One out of eight women die of breast cancer; one out of two die of heart disease or stroke.

Women tend not to acknowledge heart disease as their primary health risk and ignore instituting changes that might reduce risk. Few who smoke are quitting, and obesity is hitting new records; about 25 percent of women do no regular physical activity. Over half of all women over fifty-five have high blood pressure, and 40 percent have elevated cholesterol. A woman with diabetes is as likely to die from a heart attack as a woman who has already had one. Those with Syndrome X (35-plus-inch waist, high fat in blood, poor cholesterol levels, high blood pressure) are at significant risk.

A third of the time, a woman's heart attack is likely to go unnoticed. It is characterized frequently by pain in the neck, a feeling of ominous doom and overwhelming fatigue and/or the more familiar signs of "tightness" or discomfort in the chest, nausea, dizziness, breathlessness, perspiration, a sensation of heart fluttering or feelings of indigestion.

Were you *wondering*? Just thirty minutes of moderate activity most days, which can be done in smaller increments, dilates blood vessels, decreases resistance to blood flow, enhances HDL/LDL ratio, conditions the heart to pump more efficiently, reduces body fat, burns excess sugar, makes cells more sensitive to insulin, increases energy and fights depression, Alzheimer's and osteoporosis.

2. The fix: modifiable lifestyle risk factors

Consider this statement from the *Journal of the American Medical Association:* "Substantial evidence indicates that diets using nonhydrogenated unsaturated fats as the predominant form of dietary fat, whole grains as the main form of carbohydrate, an abundance of fruits and vegetables, and adequate omega-3 fatty acids can offer significant protection against cardiovascular heart disease. Such diets, together with regular physical activity, avoidance of smoking and maintenance of a healthy body weight, may prevent the majority of cardiovascular disease in Western populations."[8] Need we say more? Hormone replacement is not on the list.

There is no avoiding the truth that the majority of cardiovascular disease can be attributed to lifestyle choices. Clearly, what you eat, your weight and how much you move around is vital. Excess weight increases the burden on the heart. A sedentary person has twice the risk of someone who takes a thirty-minute stroll or works in her garden each day. Improvements in heart health are related to the amount of activity and not to the intensity of exercise or improvement in fitness.[9] Exercise helps people stop smoking; this is significant because one-fifth of all cardiovascular deaths are due to smoking. More than one alcoholic drink a day elevates blood pressure and triglycerides, a particular threat to women. You will lower your heart attack risk if you make positive connections with your spiritual life and with others. Feelings of loneliness, isolation and being depressed increase mortality from all causes. A person who is "heartbroken" is more likely to adopt poor health habits. Studies tell us the more optimistic you are, the more protected you are from a heart attack. And you will surely sleep better if you are in better spirits, important because not getting enough sleep increases risk.[10]

Did you know? A comparison of how high, moderate and low-fat diets affect cardiovascular risk factors showed that only people on the high-fat diet demonstrated a worsening of eight basic cardiovascular lipoprotein risk factors, even though they lost weight.[11]

the botanical/supplement connection

INTERVENTION	BENEFIT
Fish oils (omega-3)[12]	First supplement ever recommended by the American Heart Association because of its ability to reduce cardio events.
Soy isoflavones[13]	FDA approval for heart health reduces hot flashes.
Flaxseed[14]	Provides positive lipid profile.
Nuts, particularly almonds eaten daily	Improves blood lipids, homocysteine and nitric oxide ratio.[15]
Vitamin E[16]	Taking 400 IU vitamin E and 50 mg vitamin C twice daily showed no improvement and maybe slight risk, but foods high in antioxidants are not controversial and are recommended.
Tea and cocoa[17]	Contains antioxidants and flavonoids.
Calcium[18]	Improves HDL and LDL ratios.
Magnesium and potassium	Lowers blood pressure and prevents irregular heart beat.
Folate/folic acid and/or 5-formyl tetrahydrofolate (5-FTHF) and 5-methyl tetrahydrofolate (5-MTHF)	Lowers homocysteine, which injures cells that line blood vessels, and promotes coagulation; homocysteine is an independent risk factor for congestive heart failure in adults without prior heart attack.[19]
Hawthorn leaf and flower extract (*Crataegus oxyacantha*)[20]	Lowers blood pressure, reduces angina, decreases progression of atherosclerosis.
Horsechestnut seed extract (*Aesculus hippocastanum*)	Improves vessel health: "spider" veins, varicose veins; hemorrhoid improvement; interaction with warfarin.
Garlic (*Allium sativa*)[21]	Lipid modulation; reduces hypertension; antioxidant properties.
Purified policosanols[22]	Natural support for maintaining healthy blood lipid levels and platelets while promoting overall vascular health.
Coenzyme Q_{10}	Vital to cellular energy production; highly concentrated in the heart and other high-energy-requiring organs; antioxidant prevents LDL oxidation.
WHAT YOUR DOCTOR MAY SUGGEST	
Baby aspirin, one per day (81mg)	Nurses Study showed one-third lowered heart attack risk if taken from one to six times a week.[23] Ibuprofen negates aspirin's benefits.
Statins (a class of drugs that includes Lipitor, Pravachol and Zocor)	Lowers lipoproteins, although recent research suggests minimally;[24] concern over muscle degeneration that begins with muscle soreness;[25] supplementation with coenzyme Q_{10} resolves the problem;[26] lopid, while not a statin, also reduces coenzyme Q_{10}.

Keeping the brain healthy

1. The risk

About four million people in the United States have Alzheimer's disease (AD). After age sixty-five the incidence of AD (4–6 percent) increases dramatically, to 15–20 percent by age seventy and 30–40 percent by age eighty-five. The important thing to know about AD is that the sooner you are aware of the diagnosis, the greater the chance that interventions can be used to slow its progression. A delay of one to three years may make the difference in whether a person is able to stay at home.

The idea that AD cannot be diagnosed until autopsy is essentially no longer true. New imaging techniques, when combined with history and cognitive tests, result in a diagnosis with 90–95 percent accuracy—including a potential precursor to AD, a condition called *mild cognitive impairment* (MCI).[27] Just getting older and being a woman (and likely to live longer) increases your risk of AD. However, some people do have genes that make them more vulnerable, particularly for the early onset version (before fifty). Damage begins as many as twenty years before symptoms become evident.

Think about *it* ... A study done on people over sixty-five demonstrated lower cardiovascular risks in those who ate whole-grain and bran cereal regularly.[28]

2. The fix: modifiable lifestyle risk factors

The cardinal rule is that what protects your heart protects your brain. Symptoms are caused by changes in the brain, brain chemistry and death of brain cells. Inflammatory factors are at work, and it is speculated that even bacteria and viruses (cold sores) may play a part. Therefore, keeping immunity up is important. A head injury increases risk, so activities like tai chi, yoga and ballet can improve your balance and prevent falls. Always wear a helmet when biking, inline skating or skiing.

Complex thinking and writing patterns can be marvelously protective even in cases where AD-type brain damage is fairly extensive or genetic risk is high.[29] On the other hand, persons like President Ronald Reagan and the British writer Iris Murdoch prove that education is only part of the story. Staying socially active and connected to the world has been shown to reduce AD.[30] Indeed, leisure activities of all kinds—reading, playing board games, playing musical instruments and dancing—were cited as reducing dementia in a 2003 article of the *New England Journal of Medicine*.[31]

the botanical/supplement connection

INTERVENTION	BENEFIT
Colorful berries (blueberries, strawberries) and vegetables (spinach)	Anthocyanins protect brain cells' ability to respond to chemical messengers and to discourage blood clots.
Folate, B_{12}[32]	Low folate, high homocysteine is an independent risk factor for AD[33]
Ginkgo leaf extract (*Ginkgo biloba*)	Check with doctors if taking blood thinners. A recent study that reported no benefit did not use quality-control tests to determine if the gingko they were using was a clinically effective dose; you know better than that![34]
Phosphatidylserine	Keeps cell membranes open to communication, protects brain cells, stimulates acetylcholine.
Mixture of N-acetylcysteine (NAC), acetyl-L-carnitine (ALC) with B-complex	NAC enhances the production of brain glutathione (GSH) levels, central to the brain's antioxidant defense mechanisms (anti-inflammatory to brain tissue). ALC is thought to be substantially more active in the central nervous system than L-carnitine and may support energy production in brain cells.[35]
Vitamin E[36]	Antioxidant
WHAT YOUR DOCTOR MIGHT SUGGEST	
Cholinesterase inhibitor, (Aricept, Reminyl, Exelon and Cognex)	Inhibits the breakdown of acetylcholine and other neurotransmitters.
Statins	Decreases (60–73 percent) AD in those who have taken it for its cholesterol-lowering effects for heart disease;[37] unknown if statins reduce risk or if due to cholesterol lowering; statins only recommended for lipoprotein lowering.
NSAIDs (Motrin, Advil and other anti-inflammatory drugs)	Reduces inflammation, inhibits production of a protein found in plaque; effectiveness depends on two or more years of use before dementia is diagnosed.

Keeping the bones healthy

1. The risk

About half of white American women over the age of fifty can expect to suffer an osteoporotic fracture during their remaining years.[38] Osteoporosis risk increases if you have a fracture as an adult, have a first-degree relative with osteoporosis, are Caucasian or Asian, a woman, have poor health and if you have Alzheimer's.

Like everything else we have discussed in this chapter, risk increases with age. If you break your hip as an older person, your chance of mending "good-as-new" is only one-third. In fact, within a year, one-third die as a result of complications.[39] Recent research indicates that the prevalence of osteoporosis and its precursor, osteopenia, is close to 50 percent in post-menopausal women who have no symptoms.[40]

2. The fix: modifiable lifestyle risk factors

Osteoporosis is much easier to prevent than cure. Risk factors that are within your control include current cigarette smoking, low body weight, low calcium intake, too little or too much exercise and too much alcohol.

the botanical/supplement connection

INTERVENTION	BENEFIT
Calcium and magnesium	The proper calcium is so important; reread chapter thirteen.
Vitamin D	Dose of 400–800 IU is probably too low according to new research.[41]
Soy	Taking 54 mg/day of genistein significantly reduces bone loss and reabsorption and increases bone mineral density as effectively as HRT while improving lipids and hot flashes.[42]
Exercise/walking	Moderate levels of activity, including walking, substantially lower risk of hip fracture.[43]
WHAT YOUR DOCTOR MIGHT SUGGEST	
HRT	Less bone loss/lower probability of fracture—but not totally preventative;[44] low doses (estrogen and in combination with progesterone) are as effective as standard ones.[45]
Bisphosphonates	Increases bone matter density (BMD) and reduces fracture rates; new once-a-week version helps avoid esophageal/gastric damage.
Risedronate	Less stomach upset.
Raloxifene	Increases BMD (lesser degree than estrogen or bisphos-phonates); decreases vertebral, not hip fractures; four years' use reduces breast cancer risk.
Calcitonin	Inconsistent; decreases spine, not hip fractures.
Intranasal parathyroid hormone (Forteo)	Approved in 2003; first to build bone versus slowing down its breakdown; daily injection, for high risk.

Reducing your risk of breast cancer

1. The risk

An estimated 203,000 new invasive cases of breast cancer are likely to have occurred in 2002. Approximately 39,600 women with breast cancer die annually. It is the leading cause of death among women ages forty to fifty-nine.[46]

2. The fix: modifiable lifestyle risk factors

Breast cancer risk is lower if you are a vegetarian, have had (and nursed) children, are not overweight, do not drink or smoke, have less-dense breasts,[47] began periods late and have an early menopause (before age fifty-five). Obviously, not everything is in your control. A family history, more of a concern with early onset, indicates genetic susceptibility—*not* inevitability.[48] Exercise is the all-round-do-good pill that protects you from cancer![49]

As much as possible, eat organically to avoid pesticide residue, which can act like estrogen in your body. Consider exposure from dry cleaning, microwaving with polyvinyl and drinking from thin plastic bottles.

the botanical/supplement connection

INTERVENTION	BENEFIT
Foods high in antioxidant vitamins A, C and E	Ascorbic acid—particular protection for obese women;[50] helps detoxification and beneficial estrogen breakdown.
High-fiber foods and lignans (flaxseed) and a source of alpha-linolenic acid (ALA)	Low levels ALA associated with increased breast cancer.[51]
Cruciferous vegetables such as broccoli, broccolini, cauliflower, brussels sprouts, turnips, kale, green cabbage	Promotes breakdown of estrogen into good-girl estrogens.
Indole-3-carbinol	Modifies estrogen receptor activity (200–600 mg/day)
Coenzyme Q_{10}	Dose related to breast cancer regression.[52]
Quercetin and resveratrol	Polyphenols that inhibit carcinogenic estrogen break-down products.[53]
Flaxseeds	Taking 1–2 Tbsp. per day modifies estrogen receptors.
Isoflavones such as soy and kudzu	Modify estrogen receptor activity; use whole-soy foods with breast cancer; 35–50 mg daily inhibit tumor-promoting enzymes.

INTERVENTION	BENEFIT
Tea	Kills cancer cells, but not normal cells; inhibits tumor promotion, proliferation, mitotic signal transduction.
Garlic, cabbage, ginger, licorice and broccoli	Increases immunity; decreases inflammation.[54]
D-limonene oil from citrus peel	Promotes detoxification of estrogen in liver and protects breast tissue. Very safe and effective at levels >500 mg/day
WHAT YOUR DOCTOR MIGHT SUGGEST	
Tamoxifen	Black cohosh is increasingly being used with Tamoxifen for hot flash relief.

a**good** *for* **you!** *Synopsis…*

1. Have you come to terms with the reality that a "third-age" body requires some tender-loving care? You did not keep your toddler on formula, but adapted his or her diet to reflect age and biological markers. Are you willing to make adjustments?

2. How do you feel knowing that your risks for the major diseases of aging have so much of a lifestyle component? Does it make you angry? Are you in denial, feeling guilty or hopeful?

3. Does taking care of your health feel like an overwhelming task? How can you make it part of your lifestyle?

17

embracing aging naturally

Whatever a woman's definition of health, her desire is to translate it into real-life experience. Lyra and I have asked much of you in your journey of well-being. We have reminded you of just how innately capable you are. We have reassured you that you are smart enough to figure out what you need to be healthy. There is no reason to think that you cannot filter through scientific materials, see strengths and weaknesses and, in short, think critically. You can speak up to your doctor. You are an informed consumer.

Succinctly stated, we have asked you to take responsibility. How are you doing with that? Do you feel empowered and able to design a path to health that is uniquely yours? Is it possible that your experience is one of being overwhelmed and unsure? Could it be that you feel guilty and defeated?

Our hope is that you have great confidence in everything you have chosen to do, from deciding on and purchasing a natural supplement and/or herbal product to telling your physician why you are doing so. If you still feel a little shaky, take the time to reread parts of *Good for You!* Another look at what you may not have mastered is likely to make the information clear. If not, pick up other resources in your specific areas of concern.

But what do you do with the feelings of guilt over your bad health being the product of your own choices and mishandled health remedies, and the knowledge that you are indeed the master of an "ill-fated" future? You may be berating yourself with your own personal mantra: *If only I had drunk all the milk Mother kept placing before me, I wouldn't be facing a decision about whether to take Fosamax. If only I had changed jobs instead of living under tyrannical pressure, maybe I could remember my daughter's phone number. If only I had walked around the block instead of sitting in the car drinking a latté while waiting for my ten-year-old to finish her piano lesson, I might not be twenty pounds overweight. If only...*

Permit me to tell you a little secret. Even if you did all those things, there is a portion of every illness that remains out of your control. Lyra may yet get breast cancer. I may succumb to Alzheimer's disease. "Then why bother?" you ask. The answer is simple—the better your body is functioning, the greater chance you will have to be able to withstand serious and not so serious assaults to your health with energy and self-confidence. I may push back the onset of Alzheimer's to a point that I can remain at home to the end of my days without driving everyone crazy. Lyra may die with breast cancer, not from it. And should none of those dire predictions come to pass, we will be blessed with more energy and vitality for life every day we live—quality of life. In the interim, there will be time for a lot of living, traveling, playing with grandchildren, writing and, I imagine for Lyra, researching!

something to think about

HEALTH–Being able to physically do what you need and want to do—and enjoy it.

You are not a loser. You are not a failure. You are not guilty. You can do your best and make informed decisions—or not. Either way, you must simply hope (and pray) for the best. Accepting responsibility is important and can up the odds of feeling better, looking better and living longer. Emotionally beating yourself up—feeling guilty—is sure to make you sicker.

Guilt can also make you fearful of trying to get well. The reasoning is, if you fail, you have proven you are a loser or there is no hope. The more nebulous the diagnoses of what is wrong with you, such as fibromyalgia, chronic fatigue, anxiety and depression, the greater the tendency to blame yourself. But the truth is, there is no one without a burden to bear. Granted, some are bigger than others. An ovarian cancer patient described it this way to her psychiatrist:

> "I see my illness as a boulder I carry." This is not a boulder she asked to carry. This is not a boulder she created. It is a boulder she was handed—a task to carry out—not as punishment from God, but simply as part of the world's work, in the same way that some persons are handed a war in their country, and some persons are handed a childhood trauma. She has come to believe that her task is to discern

how to carry this boulder with grace and balance, how to get help in carrying it and perhaps (who knows?) how one day to be able to put this boulder down.[1]

This is taking responsibility—without guilt.

THE DESIRE "NOT TO AGE"

In an article entitled "Companies race to develop HRT alternatives" that appeared on CNN.com, Dr. Wulf Utian, head of the North American Menopause Society, is quoted as saying, "Baby boomers are a more enlightened population who are used to asking questions, but there's also almost a morbid fear of getting older. So for anyone out there who says they have a remedy for aging, there's a real potential for a short-term bonanza."[2] I beg to differ with this powerful and influential voice for women's health. I do not believe that if you are a woman aged forty to fifty-five, you have a "morbid" fear of getting older and therefore will be a sucker for anyone who suggests he owns the key to perpetual youth. You are a critical thinker and smarter than that. Hanging on to youth is decidedly unattractive; hanging on to health is not.

The best prevention of functional decline with aging is based on continuing to be as physically and mentally active as possible while fueling your body with premium nutrition. There is no money to be made in pushing such a natural, simple solution. Nevertheless, it remains the truth—and you know it. The "key" to aging well is already in your possession—embracing where you are, keeping out there and monitoring your attitude.

Pathetically clinging to youth is a waste of energy in comparison to expending that energy by enriching one's life or maximizing the impact of a lifetime of experience by sharing it with that of younger generations. However, there are a few ways of hanging on to a younger you that do make sense. Dr. Michael Roizen, author of *The Real Age Diet*, sensing the youth mania, has developed a practical approach for relating lifestyle choices to aging.[3] In fact, he has spurred development of an entire industry that relates food and other health interventions to biological aging. For example, if you are a good veggie eater—five or more servings per day—you can consider yourself two years younger (and therefore two years less close to dying or becoming feeble) than your real age. According to Dr. Roizen, you can take a full one and one-half years off your age by eating 5 ounces of nuts or three or more portions of fish weekly. If you did all the suggestions in *The Real Age Diet*, I guess you would end up in toddlerhood.

Research clearly confirms that our minds resist the negative changes of

aging when we exercise them.[4] That is why *Good for You!* asks you to
think—we know you can, and it is "good for you." Exercising your body
along with your mind will help you feel energized and less depressed, and it
will result in your being fit—not younger.

Your body does not require adoption of an extreme sport and hanging
with twenty-year-olds to be in shape. Just taking Rover for his walk will
pump additional blood to the brain, supply it with more oxygen and glucose, resulting in new capillaries and boosts in brain chemicals that are protective and strengthening of neurons and new neuronal connections. The
Framingham Heart Study found that expending two thousand calories a
week in physical activity (walking an hour per day) increased life expectancy
by two years.[5] Physical activity (only call it exercise if you want to) protects
your heart by raising cardiac output, strengthening muscle and improving
blood supply, while benefiting almost every organ and system. It promotes
increased intestinal motility, moving food along and decreasing inflammation, improving the function of the digestive system. Lower rates of cancer
and diabetes, lowered blood pressure and positive mood altering result
from staying active—no pill will do as much.

A LITTLE SUGAR TO MAKE THE MEDICINE GO DOWN

I would like to be able to tell you that my wonderful attitude, which I maintain through thick or thin, is what keeps me going despite the myriad of
health problems with which I deal continually. Unfortunately, there are too
many people around who know the truth. There have been occasions in my
life when I have been at the end of my "health" rope and so tired of
"keeping on, keeping on" that I questioned whether the effort was worth it.
All I can share is that wisdom about such matters was delayed, but not
missing—I am glad I am here. I am generally happy, despite aches, pains and
wrinkles, and I look forward to learning and experiencing new things while
relishing the old. Increasingly, I start the week anticipating new adventures,
stimulating conversations and having fun with my friends.

What makes for a good attitude? While behavioral science journals are
filled with what makes people emotionally sick, there is a dearth of research
on what makes for happiness. What is known perhaps explains my own
journey. People who feel most content in life are most often married and
have religious beliefs. Married people are happier than any other group; the
religious more so than nonreligious. The thread that binds is a sense of con-
nectedness. The basic truth is that we were made by the Great Creator for
relationship. Our lives have increased meaning and purpose when we love

and appreciate the value of others, ourselves and our God. This is what Lyra discovered was missing from her father's physical medicine. It is what brings me comfort and keeps me going when life seems too hard.

You do not have to be married to practice appreciation or love. You do have to involve your highest level of brain function to engage in loving activity. Love is a way of life—an outlook. Research indicates that appreciation is the purest, strongest form of love. It embraces optimism, courage and some place to bestow our love. Such love is outward bound and strives for nothing for oneself. It is focused on family, friends, on our work or our passions. The capacity to love makes us brave and enables us to face all kinds of everyday situations. It is a great antidote to fear. And while we love, it heals, reducing stress, enhancing creativity, relieving pain, improving immunity and reducing blood pressure.

You will not develop an appreciative and loving spirit by focusing on all that is wrong. You must instead spend time building on your strengths and blessings. If this is hard for you, let this prayer be in your mind as you swing your feet out of bed, "Thank You for another day, and show me how I can be a blessing to someone." As you brush your teeth, give thanks for your blessings—your family, friends, the work or hobbies you enjoy and the roof over your head.

I recall my mother-in-law complaining about developing sinusitis. I remember thinking to myself how fortunate she was to have lived seventy-nine years without sinus problems—I cannot remember not having it! If you cannot jog anymore, be thankful for the twenty years you were able to do such rigorous exercise, for the discipline it took and the contribution that it made to your current health. If you cannot eat some of the foods you loved in the past, be grateful for a body that knows better than you what is *good for you*. If hot flashes are waking you up, look on the time as "found time" in which you are blessed with uninterrupted time to pray. Do not waste time on your frailty or weaknesses. What do you continue to do well? How can you put your strengths to work to maximize your health or enrich life?

Contentment with life comes in recognizing we cannot always be happy. If it were easy, we would not have to struggle so to find it. Happiness is realistic. It asks us to face the truth that our career ambitions and passions for worthy causes are worth fighting, but not dying for. Our children remain a gift despite keeping us up nights wondering about their fate. Whether the pain of chemotherapy will improve quality or lengthen life remains unknown, but we march forward knowing we are doing our best for this moment in time.

Having the unrealistic expectation that every moment in life is supposed to be joyful is a recipe for unhappiness. Externals do not do it. Over 250,000 people die annually believing overindulgence and no exercise sacrificed for the pleasure of food and drink will bring happiness. The result is addiction, tolerance to pleasure, and death. Happiness is like a visitor that comes and goes. The little things deliver it most consistently: receiving a call from a friend, having the energy to take a walk, hearing birds sing or having a grandson say, "You're the coolest."

Haven't you experienced that, when you did achieve something elusive you were convinced would bring happiness, it frequently brought grief instead? *If only I were healthy, rich, married, single, had lots of kids, lived in the country...* Is your happiness waiting for an "if only"? Is an "if only" the source of pain? We live with our memories, disappointments and illnesses. We can remain stuck in them or transcend them, using them to lift us to new understanding and wisdom. Acceptance of life, contentment and happiness depends on the expectations to which we insist on clinging.

Our attitude about life is significantly tied to our perception of our choices. We do not have to repeat our family's medical or emotional heritage. We are free to educate ourselves, to choose to do it differently, to decide not to be around people or situations that diminish our emotional or physical well-being. When we choose to stay stuck, all we get for our effort is depression, anxiety, learned helplessness and illness. A happy person takes steps to make changes. There is no waiting for the good life to drop from the sky. You will not feel better unless you decide to eat better. You cannot become physically fit by just thinking about it. You will not get organized by wishing you were. It takes work.[6]

Mark Twain is quoted as saying, "Studying humor is like dissecting a frog—you may know a lot but you end up with a dead frog." Still, happiness that bubbles into laughter has much research to prove its healing effect. Laughter is a natural medicine for depression, anxiety, fear and anger. It conditions the heart muscles, exercises the diaphragm, abdominal and thoracic muscles and improves lung capacity.[7] Give yourself a prescription to laugh every day!

something *to* *think about*

HEALTH—The manifestation of appropriate intercellular response to the environment by adequate defense, cell repair and the balance of physiological function.

Religious activity and health

While some people resent that religion as a healing agent is tested by scientists, others are grateful that research is able to speak to those with doubts in a language they are most apt to hear. The National Institutes of Health is currently funding ten studies on the healing power of prayer. So far, 75 percent of such studies have demonstrated health benefits. Religion promotes fellowship, connection and positive emotions. In general, it is tied to a healthier lifestyle. There is little argument that prayer boosts morale, lowers agitation, loneliness and life dissatisfaction and enhances the ability to cope.[8]

There is evidence of a brain-immunity connection involving hormones influenced by a shift in more positive and hopeful attitudes. It has been said that faith has its own reward, but the fruit it bears is both spiritual *and* physical. Religiously active older people, those who go to services and participate in private religious activities, have lower blood pressure.[9] Research confirms that the faithful tend to lead longer lives.

IN CONCLUSION

Healthy living is not an exercise in deprivation. Once you get on the path, it is self-motivating. Today there is no excuse to not be educated. Education gives hope and knowledge to do better. The more you know, the more discerning you can be. There is, indeed, a lot of pressure to ignore one's reality, to hurry or to cut corners. Lyra and I hope that you have gleaned that being healthy requires you to set reasonable goals—that you build on small steps while focusing on what life will look like when you get past thinking that you have to have that doughnut or clean your plate. What will it take to make it important enough to change your ways, or will you wait for the crisis?

The bottom line is: You are competent and powerful; you have choices. Let others know what you need and do not need from them. "'Fess up" should you require help in overcoming blocks to getting started. It is never too late to do the right thing.

We began with the premise that, as women facing real hormone issues, our faith in the medical profession and technology has been shaken. We do indeed face unfamiliar territory, but having examined the scaffolding that once held our unexamined medical hopes and dreams, you are now aware of a defined plan (information, spiritual balance and a revitalized method of critical thinking) that will not only lead you to your personal optimal wellness, but also may influence and nurture those with whom you come into contact.

Lyra and I maintained from the beginning that we did not want to give you the fish—we want to enable you to fish for yourself. You can know what is best for you and find a health practitioner who will work with you, and you will happily discover what is *Good for You!*

EPILOGUE

temptation: more silver bullets!

aith, happiness and love aside, scientists continue the search for the next silver bullet that will enable us to remain youthful and well. The smart money is betting on the science of *genomics* to unravel the secrets to longevity by making sense of the DNA (deoxyribonucleic acid) that is contained in all one hundred trillion cells of our body. DNA is the boss that directs the chemistry that ultimately results in *you* being *you*. In a sense, the genes on a DNA strand contain "recipes" for proteins that do the work of the body. While more than 99 percent of all DNA is lined up the same in people, variations called polymorphisms make us unique and explain individual variations in susceptibility or resistance to disease (and medications). While some genetic variations inevitably lead to disease, others may or may not, depending on outside forces such as diet, toxins, hormone imbalance, bacterial exposure and so on. The potential exists for a polymorphism to "express" itself, but it is not inevitable that it will. Heart disease, Alzheimer's, breast cancer and osteoporosis are examples where disease development is dependent on the interaction between genes and environment over time. Knowing that gene expression can be influenced is opening a whole new area of prevention that one day may be individualized to you alone.

Not all current silver bullets are the result of the phenomenal information gleaned from the study of genomics. Your health food store and natural pharmacies are just as likely to come up with a quick fix as are the pharmaceutical companies. For example, at the moment, *human growth hormone* is being suggested as a silver bullet. But such faulty hype ignores the fact that a good diet and exercise will do what they are purported to do—increase lean mass and muscle—without risk. The risk/benefit profile of human growth hormone, which includes an increase in cancer, is being ignored just as it was with HRT.[1]

CRITICAL THINKING SKILLS NEEDED FOR THE FUTURE

Should anyone—a store clerk, your best friend, natural practitioner or allopathic physician—recommend a silver bullet, what are you going to do? Will you remember to ask, "Why this drug?" Do you have a condition that calls for you to consider it? Can you get the same result through adjustment of your lifestyle? What studies have been done on efficacy and safety? Who did them? For how long? Is there a botanical to use instead?

While awareness of the power of lifestyle to influence health without serious side effects is increasing, for many physicians, their practice of healing remains centered on medical technology and pharmaceuticals. As yet, training has not caught up with the new understanding of the enormous value and safety of nutrition, natural supplementation, exercise and healthy lifestyle practices in disease prevention and treatment. Change will come about when training is updated and health care is reorganized and delivered in a new fashion.

Additionally, while the population is aging, few physicians are specializing in geriatrics. If healthcare is going to be safe, timely, effective and patient centered, young physicians need to understand complex care utilizing a coordinated interdisciplinary patient-centered environment. At the moment, technical specialties are favored at the expense of patient-centered coordinated care that recognizes that older people have unique metabolisms. Palliative care must be improved so that there is comfort, dignity and meaning for patients at the end of life.

Ever since women were able to control fertility, get a good education and become more active and healthy, they have also, as the biggest users of healthcare, had considerable influence in its direction. It is the aging of the baby boomer that is the stimulus for antiaging products. But our hope is that their passion will embrace more than the futility of chasing youth. Healthy aging is a far more realistic, attainable and worthwhile goal. Work with your health practitioner to make it happen—continue to speak up! Do not settle for anything less than what is *Good for You!*

APPENDIX A

functional medicine tests

While there are an increasing number of laboratories that have functional assessments, we are including Great Smokies Diagnostic Laboratory because of their comprehensive portfolio and consistent high standards. Their direct informational telephone lines enable physicians who may be unfamiliar with their tests to speak to experts and receive information and help in the appropriate use of tests and their interpretation.

Functional assessments seek to reveal the interrelated functions of the body in order for an individualized, holistic approach to healthcare to be accomplished.

> Great Smokies Diagnostic Laboratory
> 63 Zillicoa Street
> Asheville, NC 28801-1074
> 1-800-522-4762
> www.gsdl.com

Tests most applicable to midlife women include, but are not limited to, the following:

1. Estrogen Metabolism Assessment (measures 2-OH/16-OH ratio)

2. Women's Hormonal Health Assessment (measures 2-OH/16-OH ratio, estradiol, estrone, estriol, DHEAs and free androgen)

3. Comprehensive Thyroid Assessment (TSH, fT4, fT3, reverse T3, antithyroglobulin antibodies and antithyroid peroxidase antibodies)

4. Adrenocortex Stress Profile (DHEA and cortisol)

5. Digestive Function Analysis

6. Bone Resorption Assessment

7. Comprehensive Cardiovascular Assessment (measures usual lipids and lipoproteins A and B)

8. Menopause Profile (six-day collection; estradiol, estrone, estriol, progesterone and testosterone)

9. Glucose/Insulin Tolerance Test

10. Female Hormone Profile (estradiol, progesterone and testosterone)

11. Comprehensive Female Hormone Profile (estradiol, progesterone, testosterone, cortisol, DHEA and melatonin)

12. Cardio Genomic Profile (genetic influence on blood pressure, cholesterol, inflammation and protective vitamin/nutrient metabolism)

13. Immuno Genomic Profile (genetic influence on allergy, digestive, fibromyalgia and inflammation)

APPENDIX B

dietary supplement safety

Pivotal to the safety of a botanical product is the assurance that the correct herb has been identified. Preparation is important because alterations can change efficacy and safety. Credible manufacturers will provide proof that the herb listed on a label is the herb in the formulation—they will have insisted on a "Species Voucher" or "Certificate of Origin" authorized by an on-site botanist. If purchased as a powder, a test (Thin Layer Chromatograph [TLC]) can be compared with a reference point to insure the correct herb.

Frequently, problems with an herbal product are not due to the herb but other accidental or deliberate additions. Reliable companies perform an "Adulteration Screen" to make sure no toxic chemicals (arsenic, lead, mercury and cadmium), pesticides, microorganisms or prescription medications are included. Recently, several diet products were taken off the market because they contained alprazolam and warfarin, potent prescription drugs.[1]

As of April 2001, the Office of the Inspector General of the U.S. Department of Health and Human Resources mandated that adverse events of a natural supplement company's product must be reported. A Web site (http://vm.cfsan.fda.gov/-dms/aems.html) is available for that purpose.

The Institute of Medicine National Research Council is currently reviewing ways to introduce cost-effective and scientifically based approaches to considering the safety of dietary supplements.[2] A number of agencies have begun to provide a seal of approval for dietary supplements that meet predetermined criteria.

BOTANICAL SAFETY SURVEILLANCE

Who is watching herbs, their derivatives and nutraceuticals as the industry continues to grow?

- National Toxicology Program (NTP)

- National Institutes of Health (NIH) Office of Dietary Supplements

- National Institutes of Health (NIH) Office on Women's Health

- Department of Health and Human Services (DHHS) Office of Disease Prevention and Health Promotion

- Food and Drug Administration (FDA)

- Office of Special Nutrition and the Society for the Advancement of Women's Health Research

- The American Herbal Products Association (AHPA) on the herb manufacturer side

REFERENCES FOR EDUCATING YOURSELF ABOUT BOTANICALS

- Join the American Botanical Council (ABC) and receive their esteemed quarterly journal, *HerbalGram*, for joining. Individual subscription: $50.00. Contact them at:

  American Botanical Council
  P. O. Box 144345
  Austin, TX 78714-4345
  Phone: 512-926-2345
  www.herbalgram.org

- *The Green Pharmacy: New Discoveries in Herbal Remedies for Common Diseases and Conditions From the World's Foremost Authority on Healing Arts* by James Duke, former head of the Department of Agriculture (Rodale Press, 1997).

- Education Web site of the National Institutes of Health, complementary alternative medicine resource for current research on all dietary supplements: http://nccam.nih.gov.

APPENDIX C: WOMEN'S HEALTH QUESTIONNAIRE (WHQ)

PART 1: PREMENSTRUAL COMPLAINTS

Check the symptoms you experience regularly *one to two weeks before* your period:

- ❏ Anxiety
- ❏ Irritability
- ❏ Nervous tension
- ❏ Aggressive or hostile toward family/ friends
- ❏ Engage in self-destructive behavior
- ❏ Weight gain
- ❏ Water retention
- ❏ Abdominal bloating
- ❏ Tender, swollen and/or painful breasts
- ❏ Breast lumps increase in size and tenderness
- ❏ Discharge from nipple
- ❏ Craving for sweets
- ❏ Increased appetite
- ❏ Heart palpitations
- ❏ Fatigue
- ❏ Headaches
- ❏ Shaky or clumsy
- ❏ Depressed
- ❏ Withdrawn
- ❏ Confused
- ❏ Forgetful
- ❏ Insomnia/difficulty sleeping

PART 2: MENSTRUAL COMPLAINTS

Check the symptoms and/or behaviors that occur *during your period* with a frequency or intensity that affects your daily activities:

- ❏ Cramping in lower abdomen or pelvic area
- ❏ Sharp intermittent pain
- ❏ Dull aching pain
- ❏ Upset stomach
- ❏ Diarrhea
- ❏ Nausea or vomiting
- ❏ Low backaches
- ❏ Headaches
- ❏ Difficulty concentrating
- ❏ Accident prone
- ❏ Unusual fatigue (take naps)
- ❏ Decreased productivity
- ❏ Weight gain
- ❏ Painful and/or swollen breasts
- ❏ Irritability
- ❏ Mood swings
- ❏ Depression
- ❏ Painful intercourse

PART 3: HORMONAL AND OVARIAN IMBALANCE

Check any of the following statements that *describe* your menstrual cycle, energy level or reproductive function:

- ❏ Heavy prolonged menstrual bleeding/clotting
- ❏ Menstrual bleeding that lasts longer than five days
- ❏ Absence of periods for three months or more
- ❏ Vaginal itching, burning and dryness
- ❏ Menstruation that occurs too frequently (every twenty-one to twenty-four days)
- ❏ Irregular periods (once every three to six months)
- ❏ Frequently skip periods
- ❏ Menstrual cycles every thirty-six days or longer
- ❏ Unusually light or heavy periods
- ❏ Unusually light menstrual flow ("spotting")
- ❏ Menses last three days and are light
- ❏ Bleeding or spotting between periods
- ❏ Bleeding between periods is light ("staining")
- ❏ Bleeding between periods is heavy and/or clots
- ❏ Abnormal vaginal discharge
- ❏ Frequent urination

PART 4: PERI- AND POSTMENOPAUSE

Check any of the following symptoms and/or behaviors that occur *throughout the month* with a frequency or intensity that affects your daily activities or your ability to feel good about yourself:

- ❏ Decline of vital energy and sense of well-being
- ❏ Hot flashes
- ❏ Night sweats
- ❏ Spontaneous sweating
- ❏ Chills
- ❏ Depressed
- ❏ Irritable
- ❏ Anxiety
- ❏ Anger
- ❏ Mood swings
- ❏ Headaches
- ❏ Forgetful
- ❏ Difficulty concentrating
- ❏ Difficulty sleeping
- ❏ Urinary problems
- ❏ Vaginal problems
- ❏ Dry skin
- ❏ Bleeding between periods
- ❏ Irregular periods
- ❏ Stopped menstruating
- ❏ Joint and muscle pain
- ❏ Change in sexual desire
- ❏ Difficulty with orgasm
- ❏ Painful intercourse
- ❏ Loss of muscle tone
- ❏ Vaginal bleeding any time
- ❏ Vaginal bleeding after sex
- ❏ Vaginal discharge

Copyright © 1998 Lyra Heller

NOTES

CHAPTER 1: NOW WHAT?

1. CNN.com, "Companies Race to Develop HRT Alternatives." Retrieved from Internet at www.cnn.com/2002/HEALTH/08/21/hrt.alternatives. aplindex.html.
2. Ibid.

CHAPTER 3: THE REST OF THE STORY: A NEW MEDICINE FOR NOW

1. Vital and Health Statistics From the Centers for Disease Control and Prevention, National Center of Health Statistics, Series 10, no. 194, pp. 1–98.
2. Jeffrey S. Bland, Ph.D., "Improving Health Outcomes Through Nutritional Support for Metabolic Biotransformation," 2003 Seminar Series Syllabus, Copyright © 2003, Metagenics, Inc., Metagenics Educational Programs, P. O. Box 1743, Gig Harbor, WA 98335, page 13.
3. *Taber's Cyclopedic Medical Dictionary* (Philadelphia: F. A. Davis Co, 1997).

CHAPTER 5: AVOIDING KNEE-JERK REACTIONS

1. L. Miller, "Selected Clinical Considerations Focusing on Known or Potential Drug-Herb Interactions," *Archives Internal Medicine* 158 (1998): 2200–2211.
2. More information can be found on the Web site, 4 woman.gov, The National Women's Health Information Center for the Media, Women's Health Statistics by category.

CHAPTER 6: WHEN ESTROGEN DOES WHAT IT DOES BEST

1. L. Dennerstein, et al., "A Prospective Population-Based Study of Menopausal Symptoms," *Obstet. Gynecol.* 96 (2000): 351–358.
2. J. Trabal, "Hormonal Changes Associated With Menopause," *Therapeutic Interventions in Menopause: The Role of Estrogens* (August 2000): 4.
3. C. J. Gruber, et al., "Mechanisms of Disease: Production and Actions of Estrogens," *NEJM* 346(5) (2002): 340–352.
4. Bland, "Improving Health Outcomes Through Nutritional Support for Metabolic Biotransformation."

CHAPTER 7: WHAT TURNS A GOOD GIRL BAD?

1. C. P. L. de Gardanne, Paris: Chez Mequignon, Marvis, Libraire (1821).
2. A. M. Farnham Alienist, *Neurologist* 8(582) (1887).
3. Ibid.
4. Robert Wilson, M.D., *Forever Feminine* (New York: M. Evans and Co., 1968).
5. Phyllis Fraser, ed., *Mother Goose* (New York: Simon and Schuster, 1942), 35.
6. *JAMA* 289(3) (January 15, 2003).

7. Grady D. Herrington, et al., "Cardiovascular Disease Outcomes During 6–8 Years of Hormone Therapy," Heart and Estrogen/Progestin Replacement Study Follow-up (HERS II), *JAMA* 288 (2002): 49–57.

8. Writing Group for the Women's Health Initiative Investigation, "Risks and Benefits of Estrogen Plus Progestin in Healthy Menopausal Women: Principal Results From the Women's Health Initiative Randomized Controlled Trial," *JAMA* 28 (2002): 321–333.

9. K. Johnson, "HRT Linked to Increase in Urinary Incontinence," *OBGyn News* 38(12) (June 15, 2003): 1–2.

10. W. F. Posthuma, et al., "Cardioprotective Effect of Hormone Replacement Therapy in Postmenopausal Women: Is the Evidence Biased?" *BMJ* 308(6939) (1994): 1268–9.

11. Writing Group for the Women's Health Initiative Investigation, "Risks and Benefits of Estrogen Plus Progestin in Healthy Menopausal Women: Principal Results From the Women's Health Initiative Randomized Controlled Trial."

12. *OBGyn News*, (September 15, 2002): 10.

13. Adriane Fugh-Berman, M.D. and Cynthia Pearson, "Pharmacotherapy: The Overselling of Hormone Replacement Therapy," *Pharmacotherapy* 22(9) (2002): 1205–1208, posted 10/21/2002, www.medscape.com/viewarticle/441936.

14. K. D. Setchell, "Soy Isoflavones—Benefits and Risks From Nature's Selective Estrogen Receptor Modulators (SERMS)," *J Am Coll Nutr* 10(5) (2001): 354S–362S.

15. S. J. Baek, et al., "Resveratrol Enhances the Expression of Nonsteroidal Anti-inflammatory Drug-Activated Gene (NAG1) by Increasing the Expression of p53," *Carcinogenesis* 23(3) (2002): 425–343.

16. E. T. Eng, et al., "Anti-aromatase Chemicals in Red Wine," *Ann NY Acad Sci.* 963 (2002): 239–246.

17. H. L. Bradlow, et al., "Effects of Pesticides on the Ratio of 16a/2-hydroxyestrone: A Biological Marker of Breast Cancer Risk," *Environ Health Perspect* 103 (Suppl 7) (1995):147–50.

18. P. Muti, et al., "Estrogen Metabolism and Risk of Breast Cancer: A Prospective Study of the 2:16a-hydroxestrone Ratio in Premenopausal Women and Postmenopausal Women," *Epidemiology* 11(6) (2000): 635–40.

19. S. Fan, et al., "Alcohol Stimulates Estrogen Receptor Signaling in Human Breast Cancer Cell Lines," *Cancer Res* 60(20) (2000): 5635–39.

20. T. Colborn, D. Dumanoski and J. P. Myers, *Our Stolen Future: Are We Threatening Our Fertility, Intelligence, and Survival?* (New York: Penguin Books, Dutton, 1996).

CHAPTER 8: KNOWING YOUR BASELINE

1. L. Nystrom, et al., "Long-Term Effects of Mammography Screening: Updated Overview of the Swedish Randomised Trials," *Lancet* 359 (March 16, 2002): 909–919.

2. R. P. Stolk, et al., "Ultrasound Measurements of Intra-Abdominal Fat Estimate the Metabolic Syndrome Better Than Do Measurements of Waist Circumference," *American Journal of Clinical Nutrition* 77(4) (2003): 857–860.

CHAPTER 9: TALKING TO YOUR DOCTOR

1. L. S. Picket, "Health Bulletin: 19 Minutes to a Healthier You," *Glamour Magazine* (December 2002): 109.
2. Susan Scott, *Fierce Conversations* (New York: Viking, 2002), 6.
3. Ibid., 6.
4. Ibid., 253.
5. Adapted from Craig A. Weber's seminar on communication. E-mail weberconsulting@earthlink.net or call 661-940-3309 for seminar materials on communication.
6. Ibid.
7. Susan Jacoby, "Help Yourself to Seconds," *Your Health,* AARP Bulletin (February 2003): 18.
8. Ibid.

CHAPTER 10: THE FIRST LEG—NUTRITION

1. Geoffrey Cowley, "Health for Life: A Better Way to Eat," *Newsweek* (January 20, 2003): 46.
2. Walter C. Willett, M.D., *From Eat, Drink, and Be Healthy* (New York: Simon and Schuster, 2001).
3. T. Zheng, et al., "Glutathione 2-transferase M1 and T1 Genetic Polymorphisms, Alcohol Consumption and Breast Cancer Risk," *B J Cancer* 88(1) (January 13, 2003): 58–62.
4. K. J. Mukamal, et al., "Tea Consumption and Mortality Rates After Acute Myocardial Infarction," *Circulation* 105(21) (May 28 2002): 2476–81; and J. D. Lambert and C. S. Yang, "Cancer Chemopreventative Activity and Bioavailability of Tea and Tea Polyphenols." *Mutat Res* 523–524 (February–March 2003): 201–208.
5. K. McManus, et al., "A Randomized Controlled Trial of a Moderate-Fat, Low-Energy Diet Compared With a Low Fat, Low Energy Diet for Weight Loss in Overweight Adults," *International Journal of Obesity Reat Metab Disord* 25(10) (October, 2001): 1503–11.
6. A. H. Mokdad, et al., "Prevalence of Obesity, Diabetes, and Obesity Related Health Risk Factors, 2001," *JAMA* 289(1) (2003): 76–79.
7. B. J. Rolls, "Portion Size of Food Affects Energy Intake in Normal-Weight and Overweight Men and Women," *Am J Clin Nut* 76 (2002): 1207–13.
8. J. O. Hill, et al., "Obesity and the Environment: Where Do We Go From Here?" *Science* 299(5608) (February 7, 2003): 853–5.

CHAPTER 11: THE SECOND AND THIRD LEGS—EXERCISE AND STRESS

1. Colorado University, www.coloradoonthemove.com.
2. D. Laurin and R. Verreault, "Physical Activity and Risk of Cognitive Impairment and Dementia in Elderly Persons," *Archives of Neurology* 58 (2001): 498–504.
3. K. Yaffe and D. Barnes, "A Prospective Study of Physical Activity and Cognitive Decline in Elderly Women," *Archives of Internal Medicine* 161(14) (July 23, 2001).
4. M. Irwin, et al., "Effect of Exercise on Total and Intraabdominal Body Fat in Postmenopausal Women," *JAMA* 289(3) (January 15, 2003).
5. Benjamin W. E. Wang, M.D., et al., "Postponed Development of Disability in Elderly Runners," *Archives of Internal Medicine,* 162(20) (2002): 2285–2294.
6. R. R. Wing and J. O. Hill, "Successful Weight Loss Maintenance," *Annual Review of Nutrition* 21 (2001): 323–341.
7. C. M. Stoney, et al., "Acute Psychological Stress Reduces Plasma Triglyceride Clearance," *Psychophysiology* 39(1) (2002): 80–5.
8. A. Palatnik, et al., "Double-Blind, Controlled, Crossover Trial of Inositol versus Fluvoxamine for the Treatment of Panic Disorder," *J Clin Psychopharmacol* 21(3) (June 2001): 335–9.
9. I. Cernak, et al., "Alterations in Magnesium and Oxidative Status During Chronic Emotional Stress," *Magnes Res* 13(1) (March 2000): 29–36.
10. S. E. Taylor, et al., "Female Responses to Stress: Tend and Befriend, Not Fight or Flight," *Psychological Review* 107(3) (2000): 41–429.
11. Ibid.

CHAPTER 12: AN INFORMED TRIP TO THE HEALTH FOOD STORE

1. Food and Drug Administration, Center for Food Safety and Applied Nutrition. Dietary Supplement Health and Education Act of 1994, Public Law 103–417. Retrieved from Internet at www.fda.gov/opacom/laws/dshea.html.
2. E. Guallar and Inmaculada Sanz-Gallardo, P.H.M., "Mercury, Fish Oils, and the Risk of Myocardial Infarction," *NEJM* 347(22) (2002): 1747–1754.
3. K. L. Radimer, et al., "Nonvitamin, Nonmineral Dietary Supplements: Issues and Findings From NHANES III," *J Am Diet Assoc* 100 (2000): 447–454.
4. "FTC Cracks Down on False Dietary Supplement Ads," *Am J Health Sys Pharm* 58 (2001): 1382–1384.
5. R. J. Blendon, et al., "Americans' Views on the Use and Regulation of Dietary Supplements," *Arch Intern Med* 161 (2001): 805–810.
6. A. Sarubin, *The Health Professional's Guide to Popular Dietary Supplements* (Chicago: American Dietetic Association, 2000).
7. J. Lazarou and B. Pomeranz, "Incidence of Adverse Drug Reactions in Hospitalized Patients: A Meta-Analysis of Prospective Studies," *JAMA* 279 (1998): 1200–1205.
8. *Archives of Internal Medicine* 160 (2000): 777–784.
9. A. A. Izzo and E. Ernst, "Interactions Between Herbal Medicines and

Prescribed Drugs: A Systematic Review," *Drugs* 61(15) (2001): 2163–2175.

10. U.S. Food and Drug Administration White Paper on Ephedra, "Evidence on the Safety and Effectiveness of Ephedra: Implications for Regulation," retrieved from Internet at www.fda.gov/bbs/topics/NEWS/ephedra/whitepaper.html.

CHAPTER 13: I WILL ONLY DO THIS MUCH: FOUNDATION SUPPLEMENTS

1. P. Ruegsegger, et al., "Comparison of the Treatment Effects of Ossein-hydroxyapatite Compound and Calcium Carbonate in Osteoporotic Females," *Osteoporosis Int* 5(1) (January 1995): 30–34.

2. D. D. Baird, et al., "Dietary Intervention Study to Assess Estrogenicity of Dietary Soy Among Postmenopausal Women," *J Clin Endocrinol Metab* 80 (1995): 1685–1690.

3. M. Messina, et al., "Gaining Insight Into the Health Effects of Soy but a Long Way Still to Go: Commentary on the Fourth International Symposium on the Role of Soy in Preventing and Treating Chronic Disease," *J Nutrition* 132 (2002): 547S–551S.

4. P. Albertazzi, et al., "The Effect of Dietary Soy Supplementation on Hot Flushes," *Obstet Gynecol* 91 (1998): 6–11.

5. E. D. Faure, et al., "Effects of a Standardized Soy Extract on Hot Flushes: A Multicenter, Double-Blind, Randomized, Placebo-Controlled Study," *Menopause* 9 (2002): 329–334.

6. A. L. Murkies, et al., "Dietary Flour Supplementation Decreases Postmenopausal Hot Flushes: Effect of Soy and Wheat," *Maturitas* 21 (1995): 189–195.

7. D. M. Tham, et al., "Clinical Review 97: Potential Health Benefits of Dietary Phytoestrogens: A Review of the Clinical, Epidemiological, and Mechanistic Evidence," *J Clin Endocrinol Metab* 83 (1998): 2223–2235.

8. A. R. Jeri, "The Use of an Isoflavone Supplement to Relieve Hot Flushes," *The Female Patient* 27 (August 2002): 35–37.

9. D. Lukaczer, et al., "Clinical Effects of a Proprietary Nutritional Supplement in Postmenopausal Women: A Pilot Trial," Research Report Number 113, December, 2002, 2003 Functional Medicine Research Center, the research arm of Metagenics, Inc.

CHAPTER 14: I WILL DO THIS MUCH: NATURAL RELIEF

1. M. Blumenthal, ed. *The Complete German Commission E Monographs: Therapeutic Guide to Herbal Medicines* (Austin, Tex.: American Botanical Council, 1998).

2. A. Huntley and E. Ernst, "A Systematic Review of the Safety of Black Cohosh," *Menopause: The Journal of The North American Menopause Society* 10(1) (2003): 58–64.

3. R. R. Freedman and S. Woodward, "Behavioral Treatment of Menopausal Hot Flushes; Evaluation by Ambulatory Monitoring," *Am J Obstet Gynecol* 167 (1992): 436–439.

4. N. Walsh, "Hot Flash Relief Associated With Use of Acupuncture," *OBGyn News* (January 15, 2003): 15.

5. R. Schellenberg, "Treatment for the Premenstrual Syndrome With *Agnus Castus* Fruit Extract: Prospective, Randomized, Placebo-Controlled Study," *BMJ* 322 (2001): 134–137.

6. R. Schellenberg, "Weight Loss Linked to 53 Percent Drop in Urinary Incontinence Episodes," *OBGyn News* (January 13, 2003): 16.

7. E. Boilsma and L. P. L. van de Vijver, "Human Skin Condition and Its Associations With Nutrient Concentrations in Serum and Diet," *American Journal of Clinical Nutrition* 77(2) (2003): 348–355.

8. I. K. Wiklund, et al., "Effects of a Standardized Ginseng Extract on Quality of Life and Physiological Parameters in Symptomatic Postmenopausal Women: A Double-Blind, Placebo-Controlled Trial," Swedish Alternative Medicine Group, *Int J Clin Pharmacol Res* 19 (1999): 89–99.

9. A. A. Izzo and E. Ernst, "Interactions Between Herbal Medicines and Prescribed Drugs: A Systematic Review."

10. D. Canedy, "Real Medicine or Medicine Sideshow?" *New York Times* (July 23, 1998): C1–C2.

11. K. Linde, et al., "St. John's Wort for Depression—an Overview and Meta-analysis of Randomized Clinical Trials," *BMJ* 313 (1996): 253–258.

12. D. A. Bennett Jr., et al., "Neuropharmacology of St. John's Wort (*Hypericum*)," *Ann Pharmacother* 32 (1998): 1201–1208.

13. *Lancet* 352 (September 12, 1998), 905; *Lancet* 336 (November 24, 1990), 1327.

14. Longo Leonetti, et al., *Obstet Gynecol* 94 (August 1999): 225.

15. Jeffrey Bland, Ph.D., "Position Paper: The Safety, Usefulness and Legal Status of Transdermal Natural Progesterone Cream," Metagenics, Inc., October 29, 2000.

CHAPTER 15: SHOULD I GO BACK ON, GET OFF OR GO ON HORMONE REPLACEMENT THERAPY?

1. V. M. Barnabei, et al., "Menopausal Symptoms in Older Women and the Effects of Treatment With Hormone Therapy," *Obstetrics and Gynecologists* 100 (6) (December 2002).

2. T. R. Klaenhammer and M. J. Kullen, "Selection and Design of Probiotics," *International Journal of Food Microbiology* 50 (1999): 45–57.

3. M. E. Sander and T. R. Klaenhammer, "Invited Review: The Scientific Basis of *Lactobacillus Acidophilus* NCFM Functionality As a Probiotic," *J. Dairy Science* 84 (2001): 319–331.

4. H. S. Gill, et al., "Enhancement of Immunity in the Elderly by Dietary Supplementation With the Probiotic *Bifidobacterium Lactis* HNO19," *Am J Clin Nutr* 74 (6) (2001): 833–839.

5. A. Convit, et al., "Reduced Glucose Tolerance Is Associated With Poor

Memory Performance and Hippocampal Atrophy Among Normal Elderly," *Proc Natl Acad Sci USA Reb* 18 100 (4) (2003): 2019–2022.

6. S. Worcester, "Long-Term Combined HRT May Raise Leiomyoma Risk," *OBGyn News* (November 15, 2002): 12.

7. E. A. Zerhouni, quoted in WHI, "Researchers Defend Their Findings on HRT," *OBGyn News* 37 (22) (November 15, 2002): 2.

8. Million Women Study Collaborators, "Breast Cancer and Hormone-Replacement Therapy in Million Women Study," *Lancet* 362 (2003): 419–27.

9. M. Zoler, "HRT Fails Again in Two Secondary Prevention Studies," *OBGyn News* 38(2) (January 15, 2003): 1.

10. A. Lemay, et al., "Flaxseed Dietary Supplement versus Hormone Replacement Therapy in Hypercholesterolemic Menopausal Women," *Obstetrics and Gynecology* 100 (2002): 495–504.

11. B. Jancin, "Swedish Study Ties HRT to Raised Risk of Breast Cancer," *OBGyn News* 38(3) (2003): 1, 3.

12. S. C. Clarke, et al., "A Study of Hormone Replacement Therapy in Postmenopausal Women With Ischaemic Heart Disease: The Papworth HRT Atherosclerosis Study," *Br J Obstet Gynaecol* 109 (2002): 1056–1062.

13. D. A. Schaumberg, et al., "Hormone Replacement Therapy and Dry Eye Syndrome," *JAMA* 286(17) (2001): 2114–2119.

14. L. Barclay, "Ovarian Cancer Linked to Risk of Estrogen Use," *JAMA* 288 (2002): 334–341, 368–369. Article available online at Medscape Medical News, www.medscape.com/viewarticle/438517.

15. S. A. Shumaker, et al., "Estrogen Plus Progestin and the Incidence of Dementia and Mild Cognitive Impairment in Postmenopausal Women (WHIM)," *JAMA* 289 (2003): 2651–2662.

16. A. Maclennan, et al., "Oral Estrogen Replacement Therapy versus Placebo for Hot Flushes: A Systematic Review," *Climacteric* 4 (2001): 58–74.

17. F. Kronenberg, "Hot Flashes," in R. A. Lobo, ed., *Treatment of the Postmenopausal Woman: Basic and Clinical Aspects,* second ed. (Philadelphia: Lippincott Williams and Wilkins, 1999), 157–178.

18. R. J. Santen, et al., "Treatment of Urogenital Atrophy With Low-Dose Estradiol: Preliminary Results," *Menopause* 9 (2002): 179–187.

19. T. Naessen and K. Rodriguez-Macias, "Endometrial Thickness and Uterine Diameter Not Affected by Ultra Low Doses of 17-Estradiol in Elderly Women," *Am J Obstet Gynecol* 186 (2002): 944–947.

20. M. Sullivan, "Estrogen Ring Treats Hot Flashes, Vaginal Symptoms," *OBGyn News* 38(9) (2003): 6, 9.

21. P. D. Delmas, et al., "Efficacy of Raloxifene on Vertebral Fracture Risk in Postmenopausal Women With Osteoporosis: Four Year Results From a Randomized Clinical Trial," *J Clin Endocrinol Metab* 87 (2002): 3609–3617.

22. T. Nickelsen, et al., "Differential Effects of Raloxifene and Continuous

Combined Hormone Replacement Therapy on Biochemical Markers of Cardiovascular Risk: Results From the Durolox 1 Study," *Climacteric* 4 (2001): 320–331.

23. B. S. Katzenellenbogen, "Biology and Receptor Interactions of Estriol and Estriol Derivatives in Vitro and in Vivo," *J Steroid Biochem* 20 (1984): 1033–1037.

24. J. Hays, et al., "Effects of Estrogen Plus Progestin on Health-Related Quality of Life," *NEJM* (March 17, 2003): www.nejm.org.

25. L. Dennerstein, et al., "Factors Contributing to Positive Mood During the Menopausal Transition," *J Nerv Ment Dis* 189 (2000): 84–89.

26. M. A. Hlatky, et al., "Quality-of-Life and Depressive Symptoms in Postmenopausal Women After Receiving Hormone Therapy: Results From the Heart and Estrogen/Progestin Replacement Study (HERS) Trial," *JAMA* 287 (2002): 591–597.

27. P. A. Marchbanks, et al., "Oral Contraceptives and the Risk of Breast Cancer," *N Engl J Med* 346(26) (2002): 2025–2032.

28. J. M. Schildkraut, et al., "Impact of Progestin and Estrogen Potency in Oral Contraceptives on Ovarian Cancer Risk," *J Natl Cancer Inst* 94 (2002): 32–38.

29. J. F. Randolph, "The Role of the Progestin Component of Hormone Therapy on Adverse Outcomes Associated With Long-Term Use," *Obstetrics/Gynecology Ask The Expert* (10/14/2002) Medscape Transplantation 7(2), copyright © 2002, Medscape. Retrieved from Internet at www.medscape.com/viewarticle/442195.

30. The Writing Group for the PEPI Trial, "Effects of Estrogen or Estrogen/Progestin Regimens on Heart Disease Risk Factors in Postmenopausal Women: The Postmenopausal Estrogen/Progestin Interventions (PEPI) Trial," *JAMA* 273 (1995): 199–208.

31. J. K. Dorgan, "Relation of Prediognostic Serum Estrogen and Androgen Levels to Breast Cancer Risk," *Cancer Epidemiol Biomarkers Prev* 5(7) (1996): 533–539.

CHAPTER 16: FIGHTING THE BIG RISKS WITHOUT HORMONES

1. D. von Muhlen, et al., "Postmenopausal Estrogen and Increased Risk of Clinical Osteoarthritis at the Hip, Hand, and Knee in Older Women," *J Women's Health Gend Based Med* 11 (2002): 511–518.

2. P. M. Ridker, et al., "Comparison of C-Reactive Protein and Low-Density Lipoprotein Cholesterol Levels in the Prediction of First Cardiovascular Events," *N Engl J Med* 347 (2002): 1557–1565.

3. K. Esposito, et al., "Effect of Weight Loss and Lifestyle Changes on Vascular Inflammatory Markers in Obese Women," *JAMA* 289 (2003): 1799–1804.

4. National Institutes of Arthritis, Musculoskeletal and Skin Disease, www.niams.nih.gov/hi/topics/lupus/shades/index.htm for information on lupus and www.niams.nih.gov/hi/topics/arthritis/artrhev.htm#art-d for information on arthritis.

5. CDC, "Prevalence of Disabilities and Associated Health Conditions Among Adults–United States (1999)," *Morbidity and Mortality Weekly Report* 50 (2001): 120–125.

6. D. von Muhlen, et al., "Postmenopausal Estrogen and Increased Risk of Clinical Osteoarthritis at the Hip, Hand, and Knee in Older Women."

7. N. Wenger, "How to Keep Her Heart Healthy," *Women's Health Gynecology Edition* 2(8) (October 2002): 441–447.

8. Frank B. Hu and W. C. Willett, "Optimal Diets for Prevention of Coronary Heart Disease," *JAMA* 288 (2002): 2569–2578.

9. W. E. Kraus and J. A. Houmard, "Effects of the Amount and Intensity of Exercise on Plasma Lipoproteins," *NEJM* 347(19) (2002): 1483–1492.

10. Najib T. Ayas, et al., "A Prospective Study of Sleep Duration and Coronary Heart Disease in Women," *Arch Intern Med* 163 (2003): 205–209.

11. R. M. Fleming, "The Effect of High, Moderate, and Low-Fat Diets on Weight Loss and Cardiovascular Disease Risk Factors," *Prev Cardiol* 5(3) (Summer 2002): 110–118.

12. M. L. Zoler, "Heart Association Endorses Fish Oil Supplements," *OBGyn News* (February 1, 2003): 30.

13. K. K. Hann, et al., "Benefits of Soy Isoflavone Therapeutic Regimen on Menopausal Symptoms," *Obstet Gynecol* 99 (2002): 389–394.

14. E. A. Lucas, et al., "Flaxseed Improves Lipid Profile Without Altering Biomarkers of None Metabolism in Postmenopausal Women," *J Clin Endocrinol Metab* 87 (2002): 1527–1532.

15. D. J. Jenkins, et al., "Dose Response of Almonds on Coronary Heart Disease Risk Factors: Blood Lipids, Oxidized Low-Density Lipoproteins, Lipoprotein (a), Homocysteine, and Pulmonary Nitric Oxide: A Randomized, Controlled, Crossover Trial," *Circulation* 106(11) (2002): 1327–1332.

16. D. D. Waters, et al., "Effects of Hormone Replacement Therapy and Antioxidant Vitamin Supplements on Coronary Atherosclerosis in Postmenopausal Women," *JAMA* 288 (2002): 2432–2440.

17. P. M. Kris-Etherton and C. L. Keen, "Evidence That the Antioxidant Flavonoids in Tea and Cocoa Are Beneficial for Cardiovascular Health," *Curr Opin Lipidol* 13(1) (2002): 41–49.

18. I. R. Reid, et al., "Effects of Calcium Supplementation on Serum Lipid Concentrations in Normal Older Women: A Randomized Controlled Trial," *Am J Med.* 112 (2002): 343–347.

19. Ramachandran S. Vasan, et al., "Plasma Homocysteine and Risk for Congestive Heart Failure in Adults Without Prior Myocardial Infarction," *JAMA* 289 (2003): 1251–1257.

20. W. Busse, "Standardized *Crataegus* Extract Clinical Monograph," *Quar Rev Natl Med* (Fall 1996): 189–197.

21. A. Bordia, et al., "Effect of Garlic (*Allium Sativum*) on Blood Lipids, Blood Sugar, Fibrinogen and Fibrinolytic Activity in Patients With Coronary Artery

Disease," *Prostaglandins, Leukotrienes, and Essential Fatty Acids* 58(4) (1998): 257–263.

22. L. Alcocer, et al., "A Comparative Study of Policosanol versus Acipimox in Patients With Type II Hypercholesterolemia," *Int J Tissue React* 21(3) (1999): 85–92.

23. S. M. Weisman and D. Y. Graham, "Evaluation of the Benefits and Risks of Low-Dose Aspirin in the Secondary Prevention of Cardiovascular and Cerebrovascular Events," *Arch Intern Med.* 162 (2002): 2197–2202.

24. The ALLHAT Officers and Coordinators for the ALLHAT Collaborative Research Group, "Major Outcomes in Moderately Hypercholesterolemic, Hypertensive Patients Randomized to Pravastatin vs. Usual Care," *JAMA* 288 (23) (December 18, 2002): 2998–3007.

25. P. D. Thompson, et al., "Statin-Associated Myopathy," *JAMA* 289 (2003): 1681–1690.

26. F. L. Crane, "Biochemical Functions of Coenzyme Q_{10}," *Journal of the American College of Nutrition* 20(6) (2001): 591–598.

27. Constantine G. Lyketsos, et al., "Prevalence of Neuropsychiatric Symptoms in Dementia and Mild Cognitive Impairment," *JAMA* 288 (2002): 1475–1483.

28. D. Mozaffarian, et al., "Cereal, Fruit, and Vegetable Fiber Intake and the Risk of Cardiovascular Disease in Elderly Individuals," *JAMA* 289 (2003): 1659.

29. R. S. Wilson, et al., "Premorbid Reading Activity and Patterns of Cognitive Decline in Alzheimer's Disease," *Arch Neurol* 57 (2000): 1718–1723.

30. R. Wilson, et al., "Participation in Cognitively Stimulating Activities and Risk of Incident Alzheimer's Disease," *JAMA* 287 (2002): 742–748.

31. J. Verghese, et al., "Leisure Activities and the Risk of Dementia in the Elderly," *NEJM* 348 (June 19, 2003): 2508–2516.

32. D. A. Snowdon, et al., "Serum Folate and the Severity of Atrophy of the Neocortex in Alzheimer's Disease: Findings From the Nun Study," *American Journal of Clinical Nutrition,* 71(4) (2000): 993–998.

33. S. Seshadri, et al., "Plasma Homocysteine As a Risk Factor for Dementia and Alzheimer's Disease," *NEJM* 346(7) (2002): 476–483.

34. P. R. Solomon, et al., "Ginkgo for Memory Enhancement: A Randomized Controlled Trial," *JAMA* 288 (2002): 835–840.

35. A. Carta, et al., "Acetyl-L-Carnitine and Alzheimer's Disease: Pharmacological Considerations Beyond the Cholinergic Sphere," *Ann NY Acad Sci* 695 (1993): 324–26.

36. M. J. Engelhart, et al., "Dietary Intake of Antioxidants and Risk of Alzheimer's Disease," *JAMA* 287(24) (2002): 3223–3229.

37. B. Wolozin, et al., "Decreased Prevalence of Alzheimer's Disease Associated With 3-Hydroxy-3-Methylglutaryl Coenzyme A Reductase Inhibitors," *Arch Neurol* 57 (2000): 1439–1443.

38. E. S. Siris, et al., "Identification and Fracture Outcomes of Undiagnosed Low Bone Mineral Density in Postmenopausal Women: Results From the

National Osteoporosis Risk Assessment," *JAMA* 286 (2001): 2815–2822.

39. J. A. Cauley, et al., "Risk of Mortality Following Clinical Fractures, *Osteoporosis Int* 11 (2000): 556–561.

40. Siris, et al., "Identification and Fracture Outcomes of Undiagnosed Low Bone Mineral Density in Postmenopausal Women: Results From the National Osteoporosis Risk Assessment."

41. R. Lindsay, et al., "Treating and Preventing Osteoporosis in the Wake of WHI," *OBG Management* 14(11) (2002): 90.

42. N. Morabito, et al., "Effects of Genistein and Hormone-Replacement Therapy on Bone Loss in Early Postmenopausal Women: A Randomized Double-Blind, Placebo-Controlled Study," *J Bone Mineral Res* 17 (2002): 1904–1912.

43. D. Feskanich, et al., "Walking and Leisure-Time Activity and Risk of Hip Fracture in Postmenopausal Women," *JAMA* 288 (2002): 2300–2306.

44. H. D. Nelson, et al., "Osteoporosis and Fractures in Postmenopausal Women Using Estrogen," *Arch Intern Med* 162 (2002): 2278–2284.

45. R. Lindsay, et al., "Effects of Lower Doses of Conjugated Equine Estrogens With and Without Medroxyprogesterone Acetate on Bone in Early Postmenopausal Women," *JAMA* 287 (2002): 2668–2676.

46. More information is available at www.cancer.org/docroot/stt/content/stt/ _1x_cancer_facts_figures_2002.asp.

47. N. F. Boyd, et al., "Heritability of Mammographic Density, a Risk Factor for Breast Cancer," *N Engl J Med* 347 (2002): 886–894.

48. N. A. Press, et al., "Women's Interest in Genetic Testing for Breast Cancer Susceptibility May Be Based on Unrealistic Expectations," *Am J Med Genet* 99(2) (2001): 99–110.

49. A. McTiernan, "Physical Activity and the Prevention of Breast Cancer," *Medscape Womens Health* 5(5) (September/October 2000): E1.

50. K. B. Michels, et al., "Dietary Antioxidant Vitamins, Retinol, and Breast Cancer Incidence in a Cohort Study of Swedish Women," *Int J Cancer* 91(4) (2001): 563–567.

51. V. Klein, et al., "Low Alpha-Linolenic Acid Content of Adipose Breast Tissue Is Associated With an Increased Risk of Breast Cancer," *Eur J Cancer* 36(3) (2000): 335–40.

52. K. Lockwood, et al., "Partial and Complete Regression of Breast Cancer in Patients in Relation to Dosage of Coenzyme Q_{10}," *Biochem Biophys Res Commun* 199(3) (1994): 1504–1508.

53. O. Yoko, et al., "Quercetin and Resveratrol Potently Reduce Estrogen Sulfotransferase Activity in Normal Human Mammary Epithelial Cells," *Journal of Steroid Biochemistry and Molecular Biology* 73 (2000): 265–270.

54. J. T. Pinto and R. S. Rivlin, "Antiproliferative Effects of Allium Derivatives From Garlic," *J Nutr* 131(3) (2001): 1058S–1060S.

CHAPTER 17: EMBRACING AGING NATURALLY

1. D. S. Morrow, "Not Guilty," *JAMA* 288(24) (2002): 3084–3085.
2. D. S. Morrow, "Companies Race to Develop HRT Alternatives," CNN.com. August 21, 2002.
3. M. Roizen, *Real Age* (n.p.: Cliff Street Books, 1999).
4. K. Ball, et al., "Effects of Cognitive Training Interventions With Older Adults: A Randomized Controlled Trial," *JAMA* 288 (2002): 2271–2281.
5. M. W. D'Agostino, et al., "Primary and Subsequent Coronary Risk Appraisal: New Results From the Framingham Study," *Am Heart Journal* 139 (2000): 272–281.
6. D. Baker and C. Stauth, *What Happy People Know: How the New Science of Happiness Can Change Your Life for the Better* (n.p.: Rodale, Inc., 2002).
7. C. Hassed, "How Humour Keeps You Well," *Australian Family Physician* 30(1) (2001): 25–28.
8. D. Hales, "Why Prayer Could Be Good Medicine," *Parade Magazine* (March 23, 2003): 4–5.
9. H. G. Koenig, "The Relationship Between Religious Activities and Blood Pressure in Older Adults," *International Journal of Psychiatry in Medicine* 28(2) (1998): 159–263.

EPILOGUE

1. M. R. Blackman, et al., "Growth Hormone and Sex Steroid Administration in Healthy Aged Women and Men: A Randomized Controlled Trial," *JAMA* 288 (2002): 2283–2292.

APPENDIX B

1. FDA actions can be found at FDA Medwatch: www.fda.gov/medwatch/safety.htm.
2. Proposed Framework for Evaluating the Safety of Dietary Supplements, Institute of Medicine National Research Council, National Academy Press, Washington, D.C.; www.iom.edu.

ABOUT THE AUTHOR

Mary Ann Mayo, M.A., M.F.T. has written twelve books on issues of women's and children's health and sexuality. She has appeared on the *Oprah Winfrey Show* and written about health for a number of national magazines and a newsletter. She is a charter member of the Educational Affiliates of the American College of Obstetrics and Gynecology and a licensed marriage and family therapist. Mary Ann has been married for forty years to Dr. Joseph Mayo and was his partner in establishing one of the first menopause clinics. Home is Northern California's tranquil Sonoma County where she grows lavender and grapes.

Contact:
Mary Ann Mayo, M.A., M.F.T.
P. O. Box 1039
Geyserville, CA 95441
joseph@sonic.net
Or at www.mayo.meta-ehealth.com

ABOUT THE RESEARCHER

Lyra Heller, M.A. is an anthropologist with thirty years of experience and expertise in the area of complementary alternative medicine. She is one of the founding members of Metagenics, Inc., a health sciences company based in San Clemente, California. Her life is dedicated to her family, the design of herbal products and the education of health professionals world-wide concerning the benefits and implementation of a variety of natural healing systems, ranging from homeopathy to functional medicine. In her spare time, she consults privately. Home is the Hollywood Hills where Lyra lives with her husband of twenty-six years, Richard Heller, and son, Daniel.

Contact:
Lyra Heller
lyrah@earthlink.net
www.whisperingleaves.com